Michelle R

CANCER SUCKS,
but You'll Get Through It

(Trust Me, I've Been There)

A Guide from Detection to Remission
to Getting On with Your Life

Broadleaf Books
Minneapolis

CANCER SUCKS, BUT YOU'LL GET THROUGH IT
A Guide from Detection to Remission to Getting On with Your Life

Scripture on pages 93–97 are taken from the HOLY BIBLE,
NEW INTERNATIONAL VERSION®. Copyright © 1973, 1978, 1984
International Bible Society. Used by permission of Zondervan.
All rights reserved.
Scripture quotation on page 93 is from The Living Bible. The Living Bible
was published by Tyndale House Publishers, Copyright © 1971 by Tyndale
House Publishers, Wheaton, Illinois 60187. All rights reserved.
Scripture marked as "(CEV)" on page 94 is taken from the Contemporary English
Version, Copyright © 1995 by American Bible Society.
Used by permission.
"CancerCare's Ten Tips for Communicating with Your Children," on
pages 118–120, reprinted with permission of CancerCare, Inc.
"The Most Important Rules for Cancer Patients," on pages 17–18,
used by permission, Health Care Communications.
Grateful acknowledgment to Emily Hollenberg and the University
of Michigan Comprehensive Cancer Center for permission to reprint
"Six Ways to Know Your Doctor Is an Oncologist" (pages 112–113)
and "Positive Things about Not Having Hair" (page 113).

Library of Congress Cataloging-in-Publication Data

Names: Rapkin, Michelle, author.
Title: Cancer sucks, but you'll get through it : a guide from detection
   to remission to getting on with your life / Michelle Rapkin.
Other titles: Any Day With Hair Is a Good Day
Description: [Minneapolis] : Broadleaf Books, [2024] | Includes index.
Identifiers: LCCN 2023025896 (print) | LCCN 2023025897 (ebook) | ISBN
   9781506496481 (paperback) | ISBN 9781506496498 (ebook)
Subjects: LCSH: Cancer—Popular works. | Cancer—Psychological
   aspects—Popular works. | Cancer—Patients—Rehabilitation—Popular
   works. | Rapkin, Michelle.
Classification: LCC RC263 .R34 2024 (print) | LCC RC263 (ebook) | DDC
   362.196/9940092—dc23/eng/20230728
LC record available at https://lccn.loc.gov/2023025896
LC ebook record available at https://lccn.loc.gov/2023025897

Cover design: 1517 Media

Print ISBN: 978-1-5064-9648-1
eBook ISBN: 978-1-5064-9649-8

This book is dedicated to
Dr. David Berman
and
Dr. Michael Levitt,
my angels.

Contents

Introduction

I've had cancer—three times—so I think I understand a lot of what you're feeling. Let me guess. I'll tell you how it made me feel, and you be the judge.

When I first heard my doctor utter the words "It may be cancer," I felt like all of a sudden I was underwater and surrounded by a fog of heavy seaweed. My body got a little numb, and I hoped maybe I'd heard him wrong. But he just kept talking. I don't think I heard anything except "Blah blah *tests* blah blah blah **cancer**." Deeper fog. Then a million questions. What kind? Will I need surgery? Will I need chemo? How can this be? How will I get through this? What now? I'm not ready to die.

My first diagnosis came in 2000: non-Hodgkin lymphoma, the aggressive kind. Nearly a year after surgery and chemotherapy, I went into remission and stayed there for fifteen years. In fact, my doctors pronounced me cured, though they warned me that once you've had cancer, from then on, you're technically "in remission with no evidence of disease" (otherwise known as NED).

By the time my cancer returned in 2016, it had been gone so long that when I was being tested for worrisome symptoms, I forgot to tell the new doctor that I'd had cancer. As soon as I told him, he ordered more tests. A little later, he told me he was almost positive my lymphoma had returned. And there I was . . . back underwater.

Today, after two recurrences, I'm in my fifth year of remission from my third bout of cancer. Over the last twenty-four years, I've learned a lot about having cancer, fighting cancer, and coming out on the other side. Family and friends were a support and a blessing; my doctors were amazing—well, most of them. Some things I learned from my own experience. And I've learned from many others who also found themselves in the land of cancer and had shared their own lessons with me, hard-won knowledge ranging from how to deal with nasty side effects to shifts in their attitude, priorities, faith, and lifestyle. I want to share that knowledge with you so that you don't have to reinvent the wheel or feel alone. After all, we've got to stick together!

Cancer is so limited . . .

> *It cannot cripple love,*
> *It cannot shatter hope,*
> *It cannot corrode faith,*
> *It cannot eat away peace,*
> *It cannot invade the soul,*
> *It cannot reduce eternal life,*
> *It cannot quench the spirit.*

—Author unknown

1

Just Diagnosed

You're braver than you believe, stronger than
you seem and smarter than you think.
—A. A. Milne, *Winnie-the-Pooh*

Welcome to the club to which no one applies for membership. It has local chapters in every town and includes men and women, adults and children. There are more than two hundred types of cancer, and one in three women will be diagnosed with cancer in her lifetime, as will one in two men. There are no criteria for membership except lousy luck. I know you can't wait to cancel your membership.

In just the last few years, there have been great advances in the detection and treatment of cancer, and they are making a huge impact on people's lives. Radiation for breast cancer once routinely involved at least twenty days in a row of radiation treatments. Today, shorter, more condensed courses of radiation have in many cases reduced the number of treatments by as much as half, particularly for people with early-stage breast cancer. Targeted immunotherapies go directly to the cancer site and kill cells instead of chemotherapy, which attacks virtually the whole body. CAR T-cell therapy uses genetically altered immune cells from the patient's body to attack and kill cancer. Those cells continue to replicate themselves and scan for cancer cells long after the actual treatment is over.

I'm living proof that these new treatments are leading to more NED (no evidence of disease) results, longer remissions, and added years of healthy life. When my cancer appeared for the third time, no conventional chemotherapies were available to me. I spent significant time trying to wrap my head around the fact that I had run out of resources. But in the space of one year, I was given a CAR-T infusion protocol as well as a new immunotherapy treatment, and here I am—five years later!

So take it from me: *there is hope.*

Hopefully, after your treatment is over and you have the scan that will show the results, your oncologist will say the words every cancer patient wants to hear: "No evidence of disease." But right now you probably have tons of questions and feel a little lost or very lost. *What now?* you wonder.

Hurry Up and Wait

In the movies, when somebody is diagnosed with cancer, the medical team springs into immediate action; the patient is whisked off to the hospital, and the whirlwind of treatment begins so quickly that somebody usually has to bring a robe and slippers from home. The medical team is all on board from the get-go, and they work together like a well-oiled machine.

In the real world, on the other hand, things don't happen nearly that quickly. More often, the scene looks something like this. A test comes back to your doctor with abnormal (atypical) results, so he orders more tests. It may take a few days to schedule the tests, and then a few more days—maybe even a week—to get the results. Because there are often several types of a single kind of cancer—for example, there are more than eight types of colon cancer—it can take even more tests, and waiting, to pin down the exact diagnosis.

Many people, including me, say this phase is one of the most difficult parts of their whole cancer experience. That may sound strange, but it's really true: Not *knowing* is one of the hardest places to be. Once we know *where we are*, we can start making decisions about *where we want to go* and *how we will get there*.

So try to take some comfort in knowing that right now, you're accomplishing some of the hardest work you'll have

Once we know where we are, we can start making decisions about where we want to go and how we will get there.

to do during this entire process. And ask your doctor how long it will take for all the results to come in and when you can expect to learn the final diagnosis. Typically, it takes from one to two weeks. So much for the movies.

It took about two weeks of not knowing before my first diagnosis. During that time, one of the best things I did was to refrain from telling anyone except my husband what was happening. First of all, I could hardly believe it myself. I needed time to process the possibility on my own. On a practical level, it was important to me not to make more work for myself if indeed I did learn it was cancer. Why worry others unnecessarily? Moreover, why would you want to field calls and texts from well-meaning friends who want to know what's happening? The first part of taking power in my cancer trek was being in control of when, where, how, and with whom I wanted to share the news. It saved me a lot of energy and time just when I'd need it most.

Don't Waste Two Good Weeks

Those two weeks of waiting were very difficult, but I realized something that made them a bit easier. I was inclined to let my imagination spin out into the future, and everything I saw there was terrifying. It occurred to me that my worry was only making me head toward despair when, in fact, I knew nothing. I didn't know if the results of my tests would show cancer or something else that was far less life-shattering. It occurred to me that if I assumed I had cancer and spent that time wringing my hands and obsessing, I'd be wasting two weeks. If the results turned out to be positive, I'd have just added two weeks of worry to what would already be a long journey. If the results turned out to be negative, I'd have worried needlessly for two weeks. Either way, I'd have wasted two valuable weeks of my life, and the results would be the same regardless. Every time I was tempted to worry and imagine the worst, I'd remind myself not to waste valuable time and energy. Did it work every time? No, but almost!

When you start to obsess about a *what-if*, think about something else—anything else. I promise it'll help.

After all, why waste two good weeks?

Breaking the News

Okay, so if you're reading this book, I'm going to assume that you, like me, got bad news when the tests came back.

Now you have to tell others. Telling your loved ones, friends, and colleagues that you have cancer is harder than it sounded to me. I was surprised at first by just how hard it was. I think it's hard for a few reasons. For one thing, simply saying "I have cancer" out loud makes it more real; it affirms *yes, it's true*. We know it's true, but the brain is a powerful protector that doesn't admit unwelcome news easily; it resists. For another thing, when we share the news that we have cancer, it becomes an uninvited descriptor. I didn't want to be the friend who has cancer; I just wanted to be Michelle.

Whatever the reasons, sharing this new big reality isn't easy. But there are a few things you can do to ease the process. First, when you do tell your friends, say something like "Something important has come up that I need to tell you about. When is a good time for us to talk?" The last thing you want to do is gear up for the conversation and blurt something out, only to be greeted with the news that your friend has company or is at the dentist's. Be sure to find a time and place where you won't be interrupted. Go into as much or as little detail as you want. And don't feel you need to keep a stiff upper lip or underplay the facts. Caretaker that I am, I often found myself trying to protect those I was telling from getting too upset by the news. What's wrong with *that* picture?

Remember, too, that there's no good time to deliver or receive bad news. The people who care about you want to be told sooner rather than later. Some friends of mine were very upset with me because they felt I hadn't told them soon enough. They wanted to be there for me from the start, helping me and praying for me. But they got over it. I was entering a new phase where in many ways my new motto was "It's all about me."

> Remember, too, that there's no good time to deliver or receive bad news. The people who care about you want to be told sooner rather than later.

After all, if not now, when would be a better time to put your needs first?

I recommend making some notes to have in front of you for when you share the news. A few bullet points or even a short script will help you keep it short and simple. After all, you probably have quite a list of people to tell. You can say something like "I've been feeling under the weather lately, so I went to see the doctor. The tests revealed a malignancy. So I'm exploring my options now."

Tell people as much or as little as you're comfortable with. The important thing is that you're allowing those who care about you to help sustain your body and spirit, just as marathoners need the support of those who stand along the sidelines handing out water and cheering to help them cross the finish line.

Telling your employer that you have cancer has a lot of implications. While federal law states that individuals do not have to tell their employers about a cancer diagnosis or any other health complications, many people decide to inform their workplaces for very practical reasons; for example, extra time off or special accommodations may be needed during the course of treatment. If you lose your hair like I did, being bald or suddenly wearing a hat all day will definitely give you away. But many are uncomfortable sharing the news at work.

This is a very personal decision with no right or wrong answer.

But I do have two pieces of advice: If you decide to tell your employer, make sure she hears it first—and from you.

Tell her before you tell anyone else you work with, even if it's your best friend. No employer wants to hear that news from anyone else, and despite people's best intentions, word gets around. If you decide not to tell your employer, then do not tell anyone else at your company. If you do, you can pretty much count on your boss getting the news sooner or later.

Nuts and Bolts

*Do what you can, with what you
have, right where you are.*

—Theodore Roosevelt

When you're first diagnosed, you're so busy going to doctor appointments and taking medical tests that, for the most part, the only thing you have time to do is *wait*. However, there are some simple things you can do now that will serve you well throughout your treatment.

Let technology be your friend. There are many apps and websites that can help you deal with everything. They include:

APPS:

Cancer.Net Mobile is a comprehensive free site run by the American Society of Clinical Oncology that provides many helps, including organizing helps, appointment and medicine reminders, pain and insomnia logs, questions answered by an oncologist, articles, and more for free. If you only use one app, use this one.

CaringBridge allows you, or preferably someone posting on your behalf—delegate!—to keep friends and family everywhere updated about you by setting up a page for you where people who care about you can stay up-to-date on your progress. Visitors to your site must be invited to join, which ensures privacy. They can post their own messages and words of support to you. A real time-saver and free (caringbridge .org).

Create to Heal, the app and website, was implemented fifteen years ago to help people with serious disease, chronic pain, and anxiety reduce the cycles of stress and pain. Using meditation and guided imagery, visual arts, music, writing, and motion, this is creative therapy that really helps and is free (womenwithwings.org, Create to Heal app).

chemoWave allows you to track symptoms, sleep, steps, and medications for free.

Medisafe sends reminders when it's time to take medication. Free.

WEBSITES:

Cancer.net is a website run by the American Society of Clinical Oncology that provides information about a wide range of issues as they relate to cancer. Highly recommended.

Cancer.org is the American Cancer Society's website, the first one you should go to. It is comprehensive and provides the gold standard of cancer information.

CancerCare.org: Since 1944, CancerCare has been providing free support services and information from oncology professionals and experts. It offers a wealth of help and information. A series of useful booklets covering a range of topics for both patients and caregivers is available as downloads or physical booklets that you can order at no charge (1-800-813-HOPE).

National Cancer Institute Dictionary of Cancer Terms explains thousands of cancer terms clearly and simply (cancer.gov).

Red Door Community (formerly Gilda's Club) membership starts with a phone call to schedule a one-on-one meeting with a licensed clinician who will help you customize your membership. You'll get an overview of the program, including support groups, workshops, and lectures (red doorcommunity.org).

Cancer Hope Network provides free one-on-one peer support for adult cancer patients and their loved ones (cancerhopenetwork.org).

Get a notebook and designate it as your cancer notebook. It's where you will write down *all* the information you need and things you might want to remember. You can also take these notes on your phone or tablet, but be sure to create dedicated documents for your notes if you choose to use your device. Take the notebook with you everywhere; it will become a treasured possession. Buy yourself a pretty one—you'll be seeing a lot of it. The first things to write down are:

- Insurance information, including the insurer's toll-free number.

- Telephone numbers and addresses of doctors, hospitals, labs, the pharmacy, and anyone else you'll be calling over the course of your treatment.

- Medications you regularly take for other conditions, as doctors will want to know about them.

- Questions you want to ask your doctor.

Make a cancer file. Start keeping copies of all your medical records and test reports, which you'll have to ask for. You will need them when you get a second opinion. Even if you choose not to get a second opinion, you will need to keep complete files of your medical treatment from now on for everything from insurance claims to income tax deductions. Your doctor will charge a copying fee as the physical records are legally his property. These records may be on your pages on a website portal, where you can download them.

Keep notepads and pens at your bedside and around the house so you can write down questions as they come to mind. Then enter them in your cancer notebook for your next appointment.

Get a copy of your health insurance policy from your and/or your spouse's human resources department. Find out exactly what is covered.

Keep a log of all conversations and correspondence with insurers, including dates, names, and outcomes.

If possible, delegate the recordkeeping for your insurance claims to someone else. This ongoing job is more demanding than it sounds. Unless you enjoy this sort of work, try not to do it yourself.

Keep copies of every form you fill out and every document you receive. Don't throw anything away.

Keep a calendar solely dedicated to recording all cancer-related events and expenses. Be sure to add things like wigs, prostheses, meals, transportation (including gas and parking), and lodging expenses. Many things will be tax-deductible if they're not covered by insurance. Save all your receipts. The IRS can tell you exactly what is tax-deductible (www.irs.gov; 800-829-1040).

File all bills, receipts, and canceled checks.

Delegate! Delegate! Delegate anything you can to others who are more than willing to help you. Let an organized friend be in charge of organizing a schedule of others to help with doing housework, providing meals, and taking you to appointments. Let someone who loves to write be in charge of posting updates on your progress via caringbridge.org.

> Delegate anything you can to others who are more than willing to help you.

The Most Important Rules for Cancer Patients

Know your diagnosis. Insist on seeing your X-rays, lab results, CT scans, mammograms, bone scans, and MRIs. Without knowing the details of your condition, you cannot access information about the problem on your own and make informed decisions.

Be in charge. Create an equal partnership between you and your primary care physician or specialist (oncologist).

Explore your treatment options. Get the big picture and then make your treatment decision.

Ask for a second opinion. Don't be shy.

Set up your support system and keep everybody thinking positively. Social connectedness is one of the biggest factors in explaining why some patients do better with serious illness than others. Families need to be supportive of the patient's decisions—no matter what those decisions are.

Do not second-guess your health-care decisions. Don't look back. Plan ahead. Trust your instincts. *Carpe diem:* "Seize the day." Savor each opportunity. After all, today is really all that any of us has.

Life is a full-time job. Set priorities.

Acknowledge your limitations. As a result of treatment, your energy, vitality, and focus may well diminish. It's up to you to decide what's most important and how to spend your time profitably. Time will take on new meaning. Make the most of it.

—adapted from *How Not to Be My Patient* by Edward T. Creagan, MD, Mayo Clinic cancer specialist

2

You've Just Been Named CEO

You Have More Power Than You Think

When I first learned I had cancer, I was at work. It was the middle of a difficult day, and when I learned that Dr. Berman was calling, I was pleased for the welcome diversion. I don't know why it didn't occur to me that it's not a good sign when your doctor calls *you*, but it was only when I heard the devastation in his sweet voice that I realized something was wrong. He told me a routine test had yielded a troubling result and that I needed to go for more tests immediately. He'd already scheduled them.

Within an hour, I was at the medical lab, sitting in a tiny stall and wearing nothing but an ancient cotton gown that was too thin, too short, and had too many openings. I'd even had to remove my earrings. When I heard "Rapkin!" I scooted past several nurses, doctors, and lab technicians, trying to keep whatever wasn't already showing under wraps.

It wouldn't be long before I'd learn that a big part of having a serious illness is waiting: waiting until your name is called, waiting for a prescription, waiting for a medicine to take effect, waiting for your hair to fall out, waiting for it to grow back.

One of the first side effects of cancer treatment begins within minutes of being diagnosed—before surgery, radiation, or chemo. In an instant, we go from being adults who are successfully raising families, meeting obligations, and holding down demanding jobs to being half-naked bodies waiting for instructions. At the very time we need to feel that we have power and control over our lives, we feel utterly powerless. That feeling of powerlessness is the first side effect. And it's important to eradicate it as early as possible. Believe it or not, I have good news for you: you may feel powerless, but you have a lot more power than you think.

The minute you were diagnosed, you became president and chief executive officer (CEO) of a major health concern: yours.

You are the CEO of your health; in effect, you are the CEO of the team of people who will help get you through this ordeal and get on with your life. That team includes your doctors, nurses, and a host of other medical workers. You'll be hiring people to implement the treatment you need in order to get well. More on that in the ensuing chapters. The main point here is that once you've hired your doctor and his medical team, remember

> The minute you were diagnosed, you became president and chief executive officer (CEO) of a major health concern: yours. You are the CEO of your health.

that you are the CEO—you're the boss. The professionals you hire work for you. You get to ask as many questions as you want and make your decisions only after you've gotten as many answers as you need. Sounds like a big responsibility, doesn't it? And I imagine the last thing you want right now is to have *more* responsibility. In fact, you probably want to curl up in a ball and just be taken care of. You *will* be taken care of; you will be surrounded by people whose job is to get you well again. But you also need to remember that in the big picture, you're the one calling the shots and making the choices.

As CEO, you need to hire the best staff possible. You must assemble the most qualified team of experts you can find and put together an organization that is most likely to ensure the success of your business: the business of getting well and getting back to normal. This is big business. The stakes are high, and no one has more to gain or lose than you do. Getting angry or shutting down and withdrawing will only make things worse. People with cancer who are the most proactive and informed have the best results and quality of life. There are many reasons for this; a simple one is that we all feel more confident when we are actively involved in decisions that affect our lives.

Forgive me for repeating myself, but this is so important that it bears repetition. *Always* remember that as CEO, you're the boss; your staff works for you. That means your physician works for you, as do your oncologist, surgeon, and everyone else involved in your pursuit of restored health. I'm not suggesting you should be a difficult boss—far from it. Good bosses bring out the best in those who are on their team. And you'll never have a goal that's more important to achieve than you do now.

There may be times when you're not ready to make a decision because you still have questions. If you have a question, make sure you get it answered before you do decide.

> There may be times when you're not ready to make a decision because you still have questions. If you have a question, make sure you get it answered before you do decide.

It was early morning in the hospital, and I'd been asleep. Then someone at my bedside woke me up. She introduced herself as a urologist. She'd read some of my test results and wanted to do one of two possible procedures, either of which would require surgery. She described each procedure and promptly asked me which one I wanted. It wasn't even 7:00 a.m., and I wasn't even completely awake! But I was being told I needed to make a choice then and there. She was going out of town shortly and needed to do the surgery before she left.

"What does my oncologist think?" I asked. She hadn't spoken with my oncologist and didn't seem to think she needed to.

"Which operation do you want me to do?" she asked. "It needs to be done in the next couple of days."

I had been raised to follow directions. I started trying to weigh the pros and cons of each before choosing. Then it occurred to me that I didn't have to choose anything until I got more information.

"Is this an emergency?" I asked.

It wasn't, but the issue needed to be addressed, she said. Which operation did I want? She was getting impatient with me, and I felt pressured to just make a choice.

I clearly remember thinking, *Be strong, Michelle. Tell her what you really want.* Emboldened by remembering that I was in charge, I told her I wanted my oncologist to weigh in before I decided anything. Guess what? He said not to do anything. He wanted to wait until the chemo kicked in to see if it solved the issue without a procedure. Problem solved! I was so proud of myself for not caving in. I later learned from him that had I made a choice on the spot, the procedure I would have chosen would have made it impossible to start chemo right away, and time was of the essence.

After I had time to think about what had just happened, I had a new understanding of what being CEO of my own health meant. It meant I really did have power, and I had used that power wisely. I didn't make a decision simply because someone else wanted me to fit into her schedule. I put my interests first, and it hadn't been easy. My knee-jerk reaction had been to obey the doctor standing at my bedside. She wanted an answer—right away. But if I'd given her what she wanted, I would have made a big mistake. Sometimes a CEO has to make tough calls.

Who's Who?

There are a few things about navigating the world of cancer that you should know from the beginning.

For example, you're probably about to meet with a lot of different health-care professionals. Who are they, and why so many? Here's a general sequence of cancer treatment and who you'll meet along the way.

Your **primary physician** is most likely the one who first suspected cancer. He will either perform a biopsy if it's a minor procedure or send you to an **oncology surgeon**, who will do it if a complicated procedure is called for.

If surgery is required, your oncology surgeon will operate and have follow-up appointments with you until he's ready to release you from his care. That's probably the last time you'll see him. Then you will need to secure an **oncologist**. This is the person with whom you'll decide on the course of your treatment, and you'll see him regularly during treatment. Your oncologist is a lot like your primary physician except that he's only about cancer. Even after your treatment is completed, you'll return for tests anywhere from every three to six months to once a year to make sure your cancer hasn't returned. This is the person with whom you're going to have a long relationship, and that's why it's so important that you make sure to choose an oncologist who checks all your boxes. When you find the person who inspires your confidence, who is willing to take the time to answer your questions, and who listens to your concerns, that's when you'll make the hire.

You may need radiation as a sole protocol, before or after surgery, or possibly even after chemo. That's when the **radiologist** will step in, who will be referred by your oncologist. There is a raft of other people who will help you along the way. If you're going to have chemo, your **oncology nurse** will be in charge of administering the chemo. Your relationship with him will also be an important one as you'll see him even more than you see your oncologist for the course of your chemo, which could last for months. Treatments are usually given every three or four weeks, and they can last from an hour to several hours. More on that later too.

Oncology nurses are in the trenches every day, and they can be incredibly helpful. You should ask them anything about the treatment itself, including how to handle side effects and also to report any treatment-related problems you're having, from nausea to pain. Many treatment centers employ a **dietician**, who will advise you nutritionally and suggest specific things to avoid as well as eat and drink. If a dietician doesn't visit you during an infusion early on, ask your oncology nurse if one is available for a consultation. More and more hospitals employ an oncology **nurse**

navigator, who is there to offer informational resources and to help coordinate communication among your doctors. Your place of treatment also employs a **health-care social worker**, who can be great in providing emotional support or counseling, working with families to best support a patient, and working with agencies and insurance companies regarding covering costs.

Choosing Your Oncologist

Choosing your oncologist is one of the most important decisions you'll make in this whole process. Not only will this person be your first line of defense but also going to be in your life for a very long time—not only during the course of your treatment but also throughout your follow-ups, which can range from every three months to once a year for many years. This is the person with whom you're going to have a long-term relationship, so it's very important that this is someone you feel comfortable with, who inspires trust and confidence.

Your primary physician will most likely recommend one or two oncologists for you to consider hiring. You may want to begin your own search too. Ask for personal recommendations; unfortunately, these days, most people know someone who's had cancer. There's no better source than a satisfied customer.

Before you schedule an appointment, do a little homework. Find out how long this doctor has been in practice, his field of expertise, and what hospital he is affiliated with. Read the hospital's website homepage and get a bit of background. Is it a cancer center? If not, is there a cancer center near enough that you might get your care there? How far is the hospital from where you live? This is especially important when it comes to regular treatments like chemo. If the hospital is far from your home, find out if your local hospital can administer treatment in conjunction with the oncologist's affiliated hospital.

If you have any concerns about the level of your care or doubts about which treatment protocol to choose, it can't hurt to contact a cancer center to learn if it has any satellite offices or affiliations with a hospital near you. One phone call may lead you to a valuable resource that could have a huge impact on your treatment.

TOP TEN US CANCER CENTERS

1. MD Anderson Cancer Center, Houston, Texas

2. Memorial Sloan Kettering Cancer Center, New York, New York

3. Mayo Clinic, Rochester, Minnesota

4. Dana-Farber Cancer Center, Boston, Massachusetts

5. UCLA Medical Center, Los Angeles, California

6. Cleveland Clinic, Cleveland, Ohio

7. City of Hope Comprehensive Cancer Center, Duarte, California

8. University of Pennsylvania Abramson Cancer Center, Philadelphia, Pennsylvania

9. Northwestern Memorial Hospital, Chicago, Illinois

10. Siteman Cancer Center at Barnes-Jewish Hospital, St. Louis, Missouri

It's absolutely crucial that you have complete confidence in the team you hire. They will help make your fight for survival a success. Make sure you learn as much from him as you can. He will review your diagnosis, provide treatment options, and make a recommendation for your treatment.

Remember, choosing your oncologist is one of the most important decisions you'll ever make. I just said this, but it's so important that it bears repeating. Be sure to take enough time to make the best choice you possibly can. Don't let anyone hurry you unless you're told that time is absolutely of the essence. And most of the time, that isn't the case. The general consensus in the medical community is that in most cases, it's well worth the time it will take for you to decide who you'll hire.

We tend to assume that doctors possess all the qualities necessary to do a good job. In fact, the only thing their medical degrees indicate is that they're smart. That's a great start, but there's more to being a good doctor than having a diploma. It's up to you, the CEO, to decide which of your candidates possess *all* the necessary requirements to do the job well. Those qualities include responsiveness to questions, no matter how many questions you have or how silly or trivial you may fear they are. This is cancer we're talking about, and your life is at stake.

The rule of thumb I recommend is to ask yourself one question: *Does this oncologist treat me as well as I believe he'd treat his own spouse or child?* If you suspect the answer is no, that's a good sign this candidate isn't the one to hire.

> Ask yourself one question: *Does this oncologist treat me as well as I believe he'd treat his own spouse or child?*

You and your oncologist are going to have a long-term relationship—as in a lifetime. So you'd better be sure you have confidence in him and feel some rapport. You're not looking for a friend, but you do need to have a sense that this person understands you, will take your questions and concerns seriously, and is willing to take the time to make sure you understand what's going on. If you're interviewing an oncologist who obviously is pressed for time and makes you feel that you need to hurry up and leave, then do not hire him. This is your first encounter; chances are you're both on your best behavior. If this is what you're getting now, trust me: it's not going to get better.

ONCE YOU'VE MADE AN APPOINTMENT:

Check references. Ask each oncologist you interview for a list of previous or current patients. Don't worry about offending the doctor—anyone worth his salt will respect your approach. In case you think this is overkill, check out the American Cancer Society website (www.cancer.org), which recommends this too.

Ask a friend to go with you to your consultation. He or she can be an extra set of ears and can also take notes. You have a lot on your mind now and can use the backup. Perhaps most important, you can compare notes on your impressions of the oncologist.

Be sure to bring your cancer notebook (the one in which you've written down all your questions) along to all your appointments from now on. Some people record their interviews in case they're not able to read their notes, or they forget something they thought they'd remember. The oncologist will be glad to let you record your session, but do ask permission as a courtesy.

AS YOU INTERVIEW CANDIDATES AND DECIDE WHO YOU'LL HIRE AS YOUR ONCOLOGIST, REMEMBER:

- Be assertive. Don't try to change your personality. Assertive doesn't mean combative. The point is: just don't be intimidated. If there's *anything* you don't understand, ask. Remember, *you're the client.*

- Take your time, within reason, making your decision. Your doctor will tell you if time is of the essence.

- Make sure you're comfortable with the oncologist you choose, not only in terms of your treatment plan but also in the way you relate to him. If he seems to be in a rush or unwilling to answer your questions in a way that you understand, he's probably not the one for you.

- Make sure the protocol he's recommending is the one you think is the best choice based on all the information you've gotten.

QUESTIONS TO ASK POTENTIAL ONCOLOGISTS

Ask each oncologist you interview everything you want to know. Remember: you're interviewing this candidate for a big job. And you're paying him for his time. No question is too small. If there's anything you don't understand, don't move on until you do. Be sure to include the following:

What stage and phase is it? What does that indicate?
Is this an aggressive cancer?
What are my treatment options? What do you recommend and why?
What side effects should I expect?

Will the treatments you recommend make me lose my hair?

Will I need additional therapy?

Will I go through menopause as a result of my treatment?

Will I be able to have children after my treatment?

Will the treatment affect my libido?

Are there any particular problems you would want me to call you about if they were to arise?

How long do I have to make a decision on a course of treatment?

If I have chemo, what medications will be used?

After I've completed treatment, can I expect the cancer to be completely gone?

Would you plan to stay in touch with my family doctor and other physicians involved in my care?

Will I be able to contact you by email? (If the answer is yes, there may be a fee involved. Ask.)

Get a Second Opinion

Get a second opinion. When you're looking for an oncologist, it's important to get a second opinion. This cannot be stressed enough. Why? For two critical reasons. It can help ensure you get the most accurate diagnosis and the best care or perhaps a combination. A second opinion will either confirm the course of treatment that was first recommended or propose a different option. Second, you can compare the confidence/comfort levels you feel with each oncologist you're interviewing; usually this is called a *consultation*, but *interview* is much more accurate. Remember, this relationship is going to last for the rest of your life. Even after you're in remission, you'll always have follow-up appointments with your oncologist.

> A second opinion will either confirm the course of treatment that was first recommended or propose a different option.

When you make your appointment, tell them it's for a second opinion. Oncologists expect you to get a second opinion. Any job candidate knows he or she isn't the only applicant being interviewed. One sign of a good oncologist is if he suggests you get a second opinion. In fact, if he doesn't, chances are he's not the one for you. Most insurance companies cover second opinions; in fact, many require one. You *know* it's a good idea if they're willing to pay for one!

Online second opinions are available at places like Sloane Kettering Cancer Center, Dana-Farber, the Cleveland Clinic, and many other distinguished cancer facilities. With just a little online research, you can get expert opinions without leaving your home. So there's no excuse: get a second opinion! And always ask about costs first.

It's generally agreed that with the exception of extremely rare cancers or those that are exceptionally difficult to treat, two opinions are enough for you to decide what course of treatment or protocol you should embark on. At a certain point, too many options may just make you unnecessarily confused or anxious, so two consultations are probably enough.

Every oncologist who gives a second opinion will require all your test results, scans, X-rays, and other results. It can take a few days for them to be sent, so ask your doctor's office to send them as soon as you've made your appointment. It's your life—literally. Do whatever you need to be satisfied with the oncologist you hire. This is no time to be a pleaser; make the decision that pleases you.

The Hire: Making Your Decision

After you've given yourself plenty of time to decide who the best candidate for the job is, make your decision—then don't look back. Don't second-guess yourself. You gathered as much information as possible, you've weighed the criteria, and you've made the best decision you could with the information you have. Of course, CEOs often hire consultants whom they have confidence in for major decisions, and so can you: perhaps it will be your spouse or someone who has gone with you through the process. But in the final analysis, it's your decision. Call the oncologist you've chosen and start making plans to begin treatment.

Congratulations! You've just completed one of the hardest phases of the entire cancer experience. You've made it through the excruciating time between that first telephone call and your final diagnosis. You've hired the managing director of your medical team: your oncologist. This is the most important step that a CEO can take.

From now on, remember that your oncologist and everyone else on your medical team *cannot read your mind*. If there's *anything* you think they should know, you need to tell them. If something you're experiencing is causing you any anxiety, tell them. If you have pain, tell them. Ask about anything you don't understand. Nothing is too insignificant. A great deal of the success of this entire endeavor depends on you keeping everyone informed. If you have to choose between telling them too much and telling them too little, opt for too much every time. This is one situation where there's no such thing as too much information.

> Remember that your oncologist and everyone else on your medical team *cannot read your mind*. If there's *anything* you think they should know, you need to tell them.

3

Your Body

Your first treatment won't be the beginning of your regime; there are a number of things you should do before that.

For example, you should go to your dentist because once you start treatment, you'll have to avoid any dental work. Why? All that poking and prodding they do can cause your gums to bleed and make you vulnerable to infection. It will probably be a few months before you can have a dental appointment so prepare for that now.

What You Should Know before You Start Treatment

- Have your teeth cleaned and get a complete dental checkup before you start treatment and brush your teeth with a soft brush four times a day if possible. Make sure your toothpaste has no abrasives. Both chemo and radiation are hard on your teeth and can increase your chances of getting gum infections and cavities. It's also a good idea to floss more frequently than usual.

- Do not use commercial mouthwash, which contains alcohol and will dry out the tissue inside of your mouth, which has already been compromised. To make the gargle, add one teaspoon of baking soda and one teaspoon of salt per quart of water. It keeps at room temperature for twenty-four hours. Make a new batch every day. To make it simple, keep the ingredients in your bathroom.

- If you're terribly nervous before chemo or radiation sessions, feel free to ask your doctor for a sedative. Many treatment providers will be happy to give you one but probably won't think to offer it.

- Nausea is not a given during chemo anymore. New anti-nausea drugs all but obliterate nausea in many instances. If one anti-nausea drug doesn't work, ask your oncologist or oncology nurse for a different one.

To avoid infections, do the following whenever you're in public places:

- Wear a mask. Thankfully, we're no longer in a COVID-19 crisis, but that doesn't mean it's not still out there. Besides, a mask can help you avoid whatever may be in those droplets hanging around.

- Don't use other people's cell phones; they're germ factories. And be sure to clean your cell phone frequently. Better yet, get a cell phone UV sterilizer/charger. It will kill 99.9 percent of the bacteria on your phone and is quite inexpensive.

- Carry antibacterial gel with you everywhere and wash your hands frequently. Disinfecting wipes are great for surfaces such as bathroom doorknobs, faucet handles, desks, and computer keyboards.

- Carry a little bottle of homemade gargle instead of mouthwash.

- Keep tissues with you at all times; sinus drips abound.

- Drink lots of water—sixteen or more ounces—before your chemo treatment sessions. It'll help flush the medication through your veins and will protect your veins, which chemo is very hard on.

- Bring a sweater to your treatment sessions; treatment rooms are often chilly. Most facilities will provide heated blankets to help keep you warm, but you may want to bring your own fleece throw for extra coziness.

- Chemotherapy sessions tend to last several hours. Ask your oncologist or oncology nurses how long yours will last. Then come prepared to be there for a while. You might just feel like resting, but you may want to read or listen to music.

- Bring a snack or juice.

- If you're on oral medications, it's very important to take them on time—but it's easy to forget to take them. Whenever you get your prescriptions refilled, sort your pills by dose and then make labels with dosage instructions; save this information on the computer so you can print it out easily for each refill. Put the doses with the instructions in tiny zip-lock plastic bags; they can be found in craft stores. Every day, carry the bags you need in your pocket. It'll make it a lot easier to remember to take everything on time. Get an app that will remind you when it's time to take a dose.

- Don't hesitate to tell your oncology nurse or doctor if you think one of your medications, oral or intravenous, is making you feel particularly ill. If he can adjust the dose or try another drug that's just as effective, you may be spared unnecessary discomfort. Don't worry: your medical team will never give you the second-best medication in order to reduce your side effects.

What You Should Know during Treatment

MAKE FRIENDS WITH YOUR ONCOLOGY NURSE

Your oncology nurse can be an invaluable resource to you. In fact, he may be the most helpful person on a day-to-day basis on your entire medical team. For one thing, she's the one who will administer the chemo, monitor your blood cell levels, and generally know the details of your treatment better than anyone. He or she will answer most of your questions about side effects and symptoms and can give you lots of helpful tips for coping with your treatment on a daily basis. You're going to spend more time with him than with any other single member of your team. Oncology nurses tend to be extremely caring and capable; chances are you'll come to have great affection for him. It doesn't hurt, either, to bring him some candy or cookies or any token of your appreciation now and then. My motto is "never underestimate the power of chocolate."

BEWARE OF SILOS

No, I don't mean those tall structures that store grain. The health-care community has coined the term *medical / health-care silos*, and you need to be aware of them. Just as physical silos isolate grain in an impenetrable structure, medical silos spring up when you're being treated by more than one doctor or health-care facility. Each provider is focused on his or her specialty and doesn't necessarily have the big picture in view.

> The health-care community has coined the term *medical / health-care silos*, and you need to be aware of them.

Once you have more than one doctor providing care for you, you are probably the only one who knows everything that's going on simultaneously with your care. The medical community doesn't create silos on purpose; they're the result of a lot of changes in health care, including greater specialization and the tremendous pressure on doctors and nurses to get more done in less time. But the impact on you can be negative, to say the least, if a situation arises where one area of your care may have an unintended consequence in another area.

That's what happened in my earlier story of the urologist who wanted me to undergo a procedure *pronto* when the tube that carries urine to the bladder wasn't working properly. When I asked her what my oncologist's opinion was, she looked at me like I was crazy.

"I'm talking about your kidney function," she informed me, as if my question were totally irrelevant.

"But I'm here because of cancer. I need chemo. Don't you think my oncologist should know about this?" I asked.

By this time, I was really inclined to just do what she wanted. She was annoyed and impatient and made it clear that I was not cooperating. Thank God I didn't cave in. As I've said, when my oncologist was consulted, he was adamant that I decline the kidney procedure. He was pretty sure the chemo would shrink my tumor enough to remove the pressure on the compromised urine tube. And that's what happened—almost immediately.

As I thought about the bullet I'd just dodged, it occurred to me that as well as being CEO of my health, I also had the role of general contractor. It was my responsibility to make sure the plumber and the electrician talked to one another so that I wouldn't end up getting electrocuted!

Please, please, please do not be shy about making sure your health-care providers have a complete picture of what's going on with you and what treatments you're either receiving, are going to be receiving, or are asked to receive. In some cases, they will need to consult with each other, even if they don't suggest that to you.

> Use your best judgment and your role as CEO of your health to be sure that everyone is on the same bus—and that you're driving.

Use your best judgment and your role as CEO of your health to be sure that everyone is on the same bus—and that you're driving.

If You're Going to Have Surgery

Much of the time, surgery is the first step in the process of addressing cancer. Your primary care doctor will refer you to a surgeon (surgical oncologist) who has specialty training in performing biopsies and removing cancerous tumors. You'll meet with the surgeon before either of the procedures to learn more about what to expect and to have your questions answered.

QUESTIONS TO ASK YOUR SURGEON

- What kind of surgery will I have? How long does the surgery take?

- What are the chances of its success?

- What are the risks?

- Are there any alternatives to surgery?

- Exactly what will be done in the operation?

- How long will it take for me to learn the surgery results? Who will give them to me?

- What will happen if I choose not to have surgery?

- How long does it take for a full recovery? When can I return to work?

- What do the terms *clean margins, lymph node involvement*, and *pathology report* mean?

After your postsurgical follow-up visit and your surgeon determines that you're healing normally, you'll be out of his care unless any complications occur, which is rare. You'll need some time to heal before you start further treatment, if that's necessary. At least one week before surgery, stop drinking tea or coffee, smoking, or ingesting anything that's at all addictive. You don't want to be recovering from surgery and be in withdrawal at the same time. Consider the following as well:

- Get out of bed as soon as possible after your surgery; you'll save yourself a lot of pain over the rest of your recovery. Continue this after you get home while you're spending a lot of time in bed.

- Bring a sweater to the hospital; your room will probably be cold. I have no idea why, but they always are.

- Your visitors may not realize that there are many others who are coming to see you. The result is that you, just out of surgery, will become a host for several visitors each day. Don't let this become another burden. You're going to have to say something like "I appreciate your coming so much, but I think I need to take a nap now. Please come see me when I'm home again."

- Have a friend keep a list of gifts/givers you receive at the hospital so you'll know whom to thank when you're feeling better.

IF YOU'RE GOING TO HAVE A MASTECTOMY

Ask your surgical oncologist for a referral to a plastic surgeon who is an expert in reconstructive surgery, particularly if you're considering having it at the same time as the mastectomy.

Be as choosy deciding on a plastic surgeon as you were when you chose your oncologist. You're the CEO of your breasts too.

If you're considering reconstructive surgery, ask your surgeon about TRAM-flap reconstruction instead of an implant. Tissue is taken from the abdomen and moved underneath the breast area. The bonus—perhaps the only one in this whole ordeal—is a free tummy tuck. Another significant advantage over implants is that you'll have a more natural, faster recovery, and far less follow-up will be needed. Take the following steps too:

- Don't feel you need to make a decision regarding a reconstructive surgery right away. It can be performed at the same time as a mastectomy or afterward, so you can always decide to have one later.

- After surgery, when you drive, put a pillow between your body and the seatbelt; it will protect tender areas and diminish any concerns you might have about driving.

- Move your arm around as soon as you can to avoid undue pain as your muscles heal.

- When being fitted with a prosthesis, don't buy an expensive medical bra right away. "Civilian" bras are often more comfortable and considerably cheaper. If you do buy one, make sure it doesn't have an underwire.

- Buy clothes that open from the front and are roomy.

- Use a small pillow to help protect a port-a-cath as you move around.

Ask your doctor when you should begin to exercise, which exercises to do, and who can help you. Many women have had great success with the American Cancer Society's Reach to Recovery program (reach.cancer.org), which offers one-on-one visits in person or remotely with trained volunteers who are breast cancer survivors. It is also available as an app.

If You're Going to Have Radiation

For some cancers, radiation may be used before surgery to shrink the tumor, though it is usually given after treatment in order to help keep the cancer from coming back. Your oncologist will refer you to a radiologist.

If you're going to have radiation, the technician will mark the exact spot or spots to be radiated with either a washable ink marker or a tattoo. Yes, a permanent tattoo. There are pros and cons to both: a tattoo will save you time as you won't need to be measured and marked each time. And, of course, tattoos are very cool. Washable ink, on the other hand, comes off. Some people want to wear their tattoos as a badge of honor; others would rather forget the whole experience. Be sure to ask for what you want. If you don't, chances are you'll get the tattoo.

QUESTIONS TO ASK YOUR RADIATION ONCOLOGIST

- What should I expect to feel during treatment? Will it hurt?

- How long is each treatment? How many treatments will I need?

- What are the side effects, and what can I do to alleviate them?

- What should I wear to treatment?

- Can someone be with me while I'm treated?

- Are there any activities I should avoid?

- What's the final goal of the radiation? Are you trying to shrink the tumor or eradicate it?

Save Your Energy

You've now started your new full-time job, which includes spending lots of time and energy on going to doctors' appointments, chemo and radiation sessions, lab tests, and much more. Just traveling back and forth will be more time- and energy-consuming than you expect, so it's important to accept that you simply can't get as much as usual done for now. Once you acknowledge that, you'll be less stressed and able to use your time more efficiently. Here are some additional ways in which you can use your time wisely.

If you're slated to be treated at a hospital in another community, ask if you can get your treatment at a hospital close to home. Unless your protocol is highly unusual or part of a clinical trial, you'll probably be able to arrange it.

This is the time to let your fingers do the walking. Get everything delivered that can be delivered, including prescriptions and groceries. If your pharmacy doesn't deliver, call around; chances are one will. Having your groceries delivered may cost a little more, but the energy you save will more than make up for it.

If you have a top priority, then you automatically have a bottom priority. Prioritize. Make a list of every activity that doesn't need to be done, doesn't need to be done as often, or doesn't need to be done by you. Also, do the things that are most important in the morning, when you have the most energy.

Remember that *people want to help you*. Often, they simply don't know what to do. Delegate. You can make it much easier for them by telling them a couple of specific things that would be helpful to you, whether it's bringing meals or doing a load of laundry. Otherwise, you'll get industrial quantities of lasagna when you could really use something else, like liquid hand soap.

TOP TEN WAYS TO SAVE PHYSICAL AND MENTAL ENERGY

1. Say yes whenever people ask if they can do something for you because people want to help; it makes them feel more involved and useful.

2. Even if you can't think of something you need to be done for you, say, "I know there's something—I just can't think of it. Let me get back to you." If you say no too often, people will stop asking.

3. Keep running lists of everything: tasks that need to be done, questions for your oncologist, people who need to be thanked.

4. Keep pens, paper, and eyeglasses at strategic spots around the house such as the bathroom, the bedside table, the kitchen, or the den.

5. Put all the get-well cards and gifts you receive in a single box or basket. Keep track of those that you've acknowledged. You don't need to thank everyone who sends a card, though that's nice to do if you have the energy. If you can, you should acknowledge flowers and gifts. There's no deadline, so it's never too late to say thank you.

6. Cut yourself some slack. Chances are your expectations of yourself are still based on your precancer life. Since you have cancer now, it's time to let yourself off the hook for nearly everything except doing what you can to get well. Treat yourself as nicely as you would an acquaintance, and you may find you're better to yourself.

7. Pay bills electronically or by telephone.

8. Shop on the internet. I'm sure you don't need to be told this!

9. Designate a specific time to worry. When you find yourself worrying about something, write it down and save it for when your worrying is scheduled. You can give yourself a few minutes or an hour. Then you can get your worries out of the way all at once.

10. Call ahead for appointments with doctors and labs and ask if they're running on schedule; if

not, they'll probably be happy for you to come in later in the day when they're ready to see you.

Any Day with Hair Is a Good Hair Day

Not too long after I started treatment, my relationship with my body changed. Before I was diagnosed, we were one; I was my body, and it was me. But one day as I looked in the mirror, I felt like I was looking at a stranger.

Who *was* this person? I felt like my body had betrayed me. Why? What had I ever done to *it*?

As chemo progressed, my body got more and more foreign to me.

I lost my hair three times over the course of my cancer, and it was one of the hardest things to deal with throughout my entire cancer experience. It took me a long time to realize that there were reasons for this apart from just being vain, which is how I'd always judged others BC (before cancer). But I learned that losing your hair is like watching a big line being drawn in the sand, separating your old life from your new one. It's usually the first visible sign of your illness to the outside world, and it's a shock to see yourself in the mirror or as you see your reflection in a shop window. On top of that, it didn't take long to realize that anybody who saw me—even just a stranger walking down the street—knew with a glance the biggest ordeal of my life. I felt like my privacy was in tatters.

One day, it occurred to me that all those times I'd stood in front of the mirror searching for every gray hair I could find, and pulling out a few, I'd been wasting time. Yes, gray hair meant I was growing older. So what? Growing older means that we're still alive—the very thing I was battling for with everything I had.

How many times had I wished my hair was a different color or texture, straighter or curlier, thicker or thinner, when just *having* hair is such a blessing? Have you ever stopped to think about what an incredible entity hair is? When it gets wet, it takes almost no time to dry. It keeps you warm without making you hot. When the rest of your body is sweating on a hot day at the beach, chances are your head isn't, even though it's covered with thousands of strands of hair. Hair replaces itself, unlike any garments we wear. And it keeps on growing for a whole lifetime. I could go on.

But I also knew that sooner or later, hopefully sooner, my hair would grow back, maybe even better than before. And it did—much thicker! Although I hated being bald, I tried to keep in mind that while it was a much bigger price to pay than I'd wanted to pay, it was a necessary part of reaching my goal of getting rid of the cancer in my body. In the meantime, I'd need to decide how I was going to handle being bald. There was a time when I thought about these things every day. Years have passed since I last went bald, and I don't think about them much anymore. But I will never again minimize the ordeal of losing hair to cancer.

It was traumatic and an everyday reminder of what I was going through. If anyone says to you, "Don't worry;

it'll grow back," feel free to tell them that despite their good intentions, those words aren't very helpful or encouraging.

During my third round of cancer, I was treated with a new form of immunotherapy, and it didn't make me lose my hair. I can tell you that while the protocol was still grueling, my overall experience during treatment and after was easier to handle than the other two times. Physically, I was just as compromised as I'd been the first two times, but I was much better mentally and emotionally. When I thought about why that was true, I realized that even though I had just as many long infusion sessions and felt as tired, nauseous, and weak as before, I'd been spared one huge stressor: I didn't have to think about how to deal with being bald every day and every night. During the winter, I didn't need to put my cap on at night to warm my head. I didn't need to stop and think about covering my head just to go out to get milk or see a friend. Most of all, I didn't catch glimpses of myself every time I passed a mirror just to be jolted by the reminder that I was in the middle of a battle for my life. Having a full head of hair while I had cancer was easier than having cancer and being bald.

Chemo was beginning to take its toll in other ways besides taking all my hair away. My energy was diminishing, my coloring was somewhere between green and gray, and much to my shock and additional dismay, the chemo was causing me to gain weight. I was not a happy camper.

There were bright spots as well as disappointments. Frequently, I'd open the front door and find a bag of homemade goodies dropped off by a neighbor. Several evenings every week for months and months, my friend Marie would ring our doorbell, holding a delicious dinner for me and my husband between two pot holders. I hardly ever had to cook.

One day, my son-in-law's mother, Abbie, called me. She had recently battled cancer and knew all too well the challenges of going through treatment. As soon as I heard her voice, a new feeling came over me. For the first time since my diagnosis, I was talking with somebody who'd had cancer. It was like talking to a long-lost sister for the first time.

Abbie is one of the most practical, down-to-earth people I know, and shortly into our conversation, it became clear that she had no time for self-pity or swapping sad stories. Instead, she said to me, "There are a few things you need to know that will help you a lot during your treatment. Your doctor and nurses won't tell you these things because they haven't experienced chemo, so they don't know. For example, make sure you always have tissues with you. Your nose is going to start running, and you're going to think you're catching a cold or the flu. Don't worry; you're not. It isn't just the hair on your head that's gone. You'll be losing all your hair—including the hair in your nostrils. So there won't be anything to stop normal sinus drips."

What a relief that was. A nurse had already warned me about the danger of infections, and the thought of getting a cold or the flu was as frightening as the prospect of cancer had been before I actually got it. If it hadn't been for Abbie, I'd never have learned about "drippy nose syndrome," and I'd have worried needlessly about yet another lurking threat to my health. Now that I have hair again, I don't take it for granted—even the hair in my nose!

If you lose all the hair on your head, then you'll most likely lose all your hair: arm, leg, underarm, eyebrows, eyelashes, and even pubic hair. And let's not forget the hair inside your nose! That's why you should carry tissues from now on because your nose is going to start running—for months.

Don't worry if your hair doesn't start growing back as soon as you expect it to; it takes a few weeks for it to grow from the hair follicles to the top of your scalp, where it becomes visible. Your hair will start growing back about one-half inch per month.

CRYOTHERAPY / COLD CAP COOLING

I've saved the good news for last. There are now products that can help reduce hair loss during chemo.

Scalp cooling systems and cold caps use cold liquid or gel to cool the scalp and constrict blood vessels in the head. Automated cooling systems use a cap that is attached to a small computer-controlled refrigeration machine that circulates cool liquid in the cap during the entire chemo session. Currently, two cooling systems, DigniCap (FDA approved) and Paxman, are sold in the United States. They are available at some infusion centers. The Rapunzel Project, a nonprofit organization that helps people access scalp cooling systems, has a list of US treatment centers that offer them (rapunzelproject.org). Some people have successfully gotten partial reimbursement from their health insurance providers, but insurance coverage for scalp cooling isn't standard in the United States. You may need a prescription from your oncologist if you go this route.

A cheaper alternative to scalp cooling systems is the use of manual cold caps. Similar to ice packs, these caps are to be kept in a cooler with dry ice or a biomedical freezer at the chemo facility before wearing. Because thawing takes place during use, caps need to be changed every twenty to thirty minutes.

Both scalp cooling systems and cold caps can cause headaches or other discomfort, especially during the first ten minutes of treatment. Researchers report that the effectiveness of scalp cooling depends on a variety of factors, including the specific chemo regimen being used. Get your doctor's or oncology nurse's input before you make a decision.

If you do use scalp cooling, be extra gentle with your hair to prevent damage. You should

- Use a gentle shampoo.

- Avoid dyeing your hair until three months after you've completed chemo.

- Avoid using blow dryers and any other items that employ heat.

- Comb and brush your hair gently.

Success rates vary.

The Dreaded Wig: Why You Shouldn't Spend More Than Two Hundred Dollars

Because of new therapies such as immunotherapy, many people undergoing treatment do not lose their hair in the process. Thank goodness that awful side effect is no longer necessarily a given. But if you are going to lose your hair, you'll want to consider in advance how you're going to deal with it. Ask your oncologist when to expect it to fall out; usually it happens within ten to fourteen days of your first treatment, gradually at first and quite quickly after that. It's a very good idea to get your head shaved at least two or three days before then. Trust me, you don't want to wake up one morning and find handfuls of hair on your pillow or watch it all whoosh down the drain as you're shampooing it in the shower. It's even more distressing than having your head shaved. If you do choose to have your head shaved, you can ask for one-fourth to one-half of an inch of hair to be left on your head. You'll hardly notice when that hair falls out, and you'll have hair a little longer than a totally bald shave.

Be sure to keep a lock of your hair so you can use it as a reference when you're buying a wig so that you can come as close as possible to match your own color. Or you may want to throw caution to the wind and get hot pink or Marilyn Monroe blond. Even if you do, sooner or later you'll

Be sure to keep a lock of your hair so you can use it as a reference when you're buying a wig so that you can come as close as possible to match your own color.

probably want one that's your own color. Ask a friend or loved one to go with you when you have your head shaved. There are wig salons and beauty shops that will do it for you in a private area. My husband shaved my head in the privacy of our bathroom. It didn't cost a thing, and you would have thought that Oribe had done it!

Look at your hair loss as visible evidence that the chemo is in your body and doing what it's supposed to do. One woman made several small braids out of her hair, tied a ribbon at each end, and gave them to friends and loved ones with a note asking that they say a little prayer for her when they looked at them. After she went into remission, she hosted a tea for them. Ticket for admission: one braid.

Almost immediately after you lose your hair—and in some cases, before—your scalp will become itchy and painful to the touch. That's caused by the treatment. Rub liquid vitamin E on your head to soothe and relieve the irritation.

Save your receipt for your wig and ask your doctor for a prescription for a cranial prosthesis. That way, your insurance may cover the cost. If it doesn't, the wig is tax-deductible.

WIG SHOPPING

I had a hard time anticipating getting a wig. It brought home the fact that I was going to be bald for many months. It made me realize even more intensely than before that I had cancer; I hadn't imagined that was possible.

I decided to get the best wig I could possibly buy. After all, it was going to be on my head eighteen hours a day for the next several months. So I went to the best wig salon I could find. They recommended that I get one that was 100 percent human hair. The cost: one thousand dollars.

"Maybe I don't need the *very* best. Do you have anything almost as good?" I asked.

Yes, they told me, they had one made out of a combination of human and synthetic hair. It was only seven hundred dollars. I gulped and said, "I'll take it."

Some people decide this is their chance to go blond or become a redhead or a brunette for the first time, but I went with my natural color—without the gray. I also chose my traditional chin-length style. I wanted to look as much the same as possible. At first, I was so happy to have hair that I swore I'd wear it at all times, except when I was asleep. That resolution lasted about twenty minutes. Maybe I could have done it for a day or so or a week, but this was a long-term proposition. So I opted for comfort and usually went au naturel when I was at home. I already had a new empathy for men with toupees.

Shortly after I started wearing my wig, I began to pinpoint the physical discomfort I was feeling. My wig was heavier than my own hair. Heavy enough that I was aware of it all the time it was on my head. And it was hot. But there was another more uncomfortable sensation: my head was itchy. All the time. But what could I do? I assumed that was the price I had to pay in order to look like an earthling, and I'd just bear it. Which brings me to two-hundred-dollar wigs.

One day, I came across a wig store in a strip mall. It wasn't at all fancy. They didn't even have human-hair wigs. But I was desperate. My head had been hot and itchy for months, and I had months to go. I tried on a short synthetic wig. Much to my surprise, it didn't make my head hot, and it wasn't nearly as itchy as my "good" wig. That's because the saleswoman gave me a stocking cap to put on first, and that provided immediate relief. So much for the top-notch care of a fancy wig salon. Nobody *there* had told me that. The cheaper wig also weighed far less, which also made it more comfortable. On top of that, the synthetic wig looked at least as natural as my designer wig, possibly better. Even if that was just a mirage, I was definitely a lot happier and cooler. Whatever the cost, I was going to spring for it.

"How much?" I asked.

"Two hundred dollars," the saleswoman answered.

I couldn't believe my ears. "I'll take it," I said before she could change her mind.

I probably should have bought a couple more styles just for variety. I put my expensive wig in the back of a drawer and never took it out. Granted, the cheaper wig wasn't perfect. I still knew something foreign was on my head. But it was a godsend to me.

Hence my advice: Do not spend more than two hundred dollars on your wig. It will probably be far cooler and not nearly as heavy as a human-hair wig. Besides, if you

Do not spend more than two hundred dollars on your wig. decide you want to spring for a higher-quality one, you always can. If not, you won't have blown several hundred dollars on a wig that might well end up in the back of a drawer.

Since you lose 30 percent of your body heat through your head, there's a good chance you'll be chilly when you go to bed. Cotton caps designed to wear to bed are often available at wig shops or from the Tender Loving Care (TLC) catalog. This is also a great place to get modestly priced wigs, wig accessories, and more tips about wearing your wig more easily and comfortably. If possible, I recommend getting your wig at a brick-and-mortar store so you can try some on before you choose one.

The American Cancer Society has a website devoted to cancer aids, from wigs to breast forms to medical alert products, as well as wig accessories (TLC catalog: tlcdirect .org). They also have a telephone customer service line if you want to talk with someone about a product (1-800-850-9445). Their "Him Wig Collection" carries hairpieces for men who suffer from hair loss related to cancer, chemo, or alopecia.

Here are a few tips that will give you more comfort and convenience:

- Be sure to wear a wig liner, an inexpensive nylon mesh cap worn under the wig that prevents itching. I consider this the most important wig accessory to have.

- Wig shampoo is available for maintenance, though I used diluted regular shampoo, which worked just fine. Wash your wig gently about every two weeks. Wig conditioners are also available, which can help maintain style.

- Use eyeliner and eyebrow pencil and brush to "replace" thin or missing lashes and brows.

- Take a close-up headshot photo before you lose your hair so you can use it as a guide for applying your eyebrow pencil.

For a more realistic look when wearing your wig, lightly brush eyebrow pencil color along your "scalp line" before you put the wig on. It will enhance the illusion of roots under the hair.

SPEAKING OF HEADWEAR

The day came when I could no longer stand to wear a wig out all the time, especially when spring arrived. Scarves were a godsend.

Be sure to buy eighteen- or twenty-four-inch square scarves. Larger ones are too big.

The very best headwear I found was, I'm proud to say, something from the "necessity is the mother of invention" theory. I definitely had hair envy and bought every drugstore hairpiece I came across. One hot summer day, I pulled out a ponytail and sewed it on the inside through that little hole in the back of my favorite baseball cap and *voilà*—the closest thing to my natural hair look that I'd had so far! I wore that cap well after Labor Day, even if it was white. I highly recommend it.

When your hair grows back, it may be different from your original color. My formerly brown hair was replaced with gray hair.

"They gave me somebody else's hair," I said to no one in particular. "It must be a mistake."

On the other hand, a friend's hair grew in her exact former shade. If I were you, I'd assume the best, and if you do get gray hair, at least you'll have had several months expecting your normal color instead of worrying. Besides, gray hair has become a lot more popular in the last few years. The second time my hair grew back, it appeared as a resplendent mix of colors ranging from black to white; now it's one of my best features.

Coping with Side Effects

Fortunately for us, medical research has come up with anticancer drugs and treatments that have far fewer side effects than they did even a few years ago. Granted, there's still a long way to go, but people who are undergoing treatment today are actually fortunate that science has come such a long way. The list of side effects that follows is pretty comprehensive, and few people experience all of them, so don't get nervous when you read this section.

NAUSEA

Unfortunately, nausea is a common side effect of chemo. But there's good news: many powerful anti-nausea drugs have been developed in the last few years that can help relieve or even nearly eliminate it much of the time. And there are many of them. So if one doesn't work for you, ask your oncology nurse or oncologist for a different one.

One of the very best remedies I found for all but the worst nausea was a sample candy I picked up at my oncologist's office: Prince of Peace Mango Ginger Chews, individually wrapped all-natural candies that taste great and really did the trick for me.

TIPS FOR COPING WITH NAUSEA

Ask your doctor or oncology nurse for nausea medication.

Invest in a big fluffy dog bed for the bathroom if you find yourself there for long periods of time. Nicer to lie on than the cold, hard floor.

Eat a snack or a light meal before you have your chemo or radiation treatment to help prevent nausea.

At the very first sign of nausea, take your anti-nausea medication. The longer you put it off, the harder it will be for it to take effect.

Try to keep eating—something. Even just a cracker. It's important to get nutrition both to fuel your body and also to keep your body metabolizing your medications.

Eat small amounts often during the day instead of having three larger meals.

Eat bland carbs such as mashed potatoes, crackers, and rice.

Suck on flavored ice pops when you get bored with ice chips.

Help stimulate your appetite by drinking a small glass of port or wine about half an hour before a meal.

Don't drink anything with your meals; drink before or after meals.

Drink ginger ale, ginger tea, or other ginger products—they help ease nausea.

Suck on Prince of Peace Mango Ginger Chews (available on the web and in some retail stores). Keep a couple in your purse.

Eat very slowly; chew each mouthful thirty times before you swallow.

Eat foods that are room temperature or cold.

Call the doctor if your nausea and vomiting last for more than two days.

Use scent-free products, such as deodorants and lotions, as much as possible to prevent odor-induced nausea.

FATIGUE

One very subtle but real side effect of radiation is what *doesn't* happen as a result of it. Because radiation doesn't cause complete hair loss, you probably don't "look sick." So people often forget you're fighting for your life and don't have much energy to do a whole lot else. They don't mean to, but they often expect more from you than they would if you were bald or green. This is actually one of the worst things about fatigue: it's invisible.

There are other signs of fatigue along with feeling drained and listless, including being irritable and having difficulty concentrating, talking, and making decisions. When you feel these, slow down and rest.

Take several brief power naps or rest breaks a day instead of one long one. They'll actually promote healing as well as raise your energy level.

Try to do activities that you enjoy but shorten their length. That way, you'll feel less deprived. Light exercise helps to relieve fatigue.

Drink decaf beverages; surprisingly, too much caffeine depletes your energy.

Rest whenever you need to. This is not the time to be polite or a hostess or responsible for entertainment. Don't feel guilty about telling those around you that you're going to rest. They can continue their visit among themselves.

Eat protein. It helps rebuild muscle strength.

This may sound counterintuitive, but try to take a walk daily, even a short one. Researchers have found that a walking routine improves fatigue for those undergoing cancer treatment.

NOSE, MOUTH, AND THROAT IRRITATION

Many people who have chemo or radiation experience inflammation inside the nose and throat. Here are some ways to soothe this condition:

Keep your mouth clean and moist. Don't use commercial mouthwashes, which usually contain alcohol. Alcohol dries out the inside of your mouth, which may well already be dry from medications.

Use a mixture of baking soda or salt with warm water instead.

Avoid acidic foods and juices such as orange, tomato, and grapefruit.

SKIN IRRITATION/DISCOLORATION

If you're having radiation, your skin will probably begin to look sunburned or even tanned where it's been radiated. It may even appear discolored. If it does, don't worry; that will go away. You can expect your skin to become tender and possibly itchy. Here are some ways to prevent or at least alleviate discomfort:

Be sure to use deodorants that do not contain aluminum. Good ones include Tom's of Maine, unscented Dove, or natural crystal deodorants, which are easily found in any drugstore. A much cheaper and equally effective solution is to put pure cornstarch in an old spice shaker.

Ask your radiation provider for a cream designed to reduce your symptoms.

Use lukewarm water and mild soap to wash and pat your skin dry.

Don't use heating pads or ice packs on your skin.

Don't use any skin lotions for at least two hours after your treatment.

Don't expose your treated skin to the sun.

HAND-FOOT SYNDROME

Hand-foot syndrome is a skin reaction to some kinds of chemo; its symptoms include reddish hands and feet, swelling, and burning or tingling sensations. To help relieve it, try the following:

Use fragrance-free skin care creams such as Aquaphor or Cetaphil.

Before you go to bed, apply the cream to your hands and/or feet and wear cotton gloves and cotton socks to bed. This will ensure that the cream is absorbed rather than rubbed off while you sleep.

Use ice packs, gel ice packs, or even a bag of frozen vegetables—peas are best—to help relieve pain.

Try taking a cool, not cold, bath.

Don't wash dishes—hot water aggravates the skin.

If you must wash dishes, don't wear rubber gloves; they'll act like a greenhouse on your skin. You'll just have to do without. Better yet, get someone else to do your dishes.

Stay out of the sun as much as possible.

NEUROPATHY

Some cancer treatments cause peripheral neuropathy, which is damage to the nerves in your hands and feet. The most common symptoms include tingling, pins and needles, numbness, or other sensations; some people experience pain. In most cases, all of these side effects will gradually decline or go away completely after treatment. Tell your oncologist / oncology nurse if you're experiencing this and any other side effects.

Cryotherapy, or cold therapy, has been shown to reduce neuropathy. Special socks and gloves that use cooling gel and/or ice can be worn during treatment to reduce nerve damage and relieve discomfort. They're much cheaper and simpler to use than cold caps used to reduce hair loss. Costs for socks, gloves, and cold packs range from about fifteen to thirty-five dollars per item. I used these during my chemo sessions, and while I'm not sure what I avoided, they did seem to slow down the nerve damage, and additional symptoms seemed to be less intense than before I started using them.

INSOMNIA

When you have laboriously accomplished your daily task, go to sleep in Peace. God is awake.
—Victor Hugo

Another great irony of cancer is that just when you need your rest the most, insomnia often strikes, thanks to some of the fine ingredients in your treatment cocktail. If you're taking steroids, they'll probably make you wake up in the night, full of the kind of antsy energy that makes you want to clean your house from top to bottom. If that happens and you really want to clean, go for it. Enjoy the energy because the time will come when you wish you had it!

Chemo may well cause insomnia, too, but unlike that from steroids, you'll be awake and tired. I woke up in the early-morning hours almost daily during my chemo. Once I realized that I couldn't make myself go back to sleep, I started going into another room where I kept a blanket, pillow, crossword puzzles, many magazines, stationery, a radio, and a TV. Usually, one of those things would get my attention, and then I'd go with the flow, not worrying about how long I was going to stay awake. Sometimes I'd get tired after ten minutes; other times it took two hours to get back to sleep.

Other people with insomnia have found these things helpful:

- Don't take naps during the day, no matter how tired you are.

- Use your bed for two things: sleep and sex. Find another place for all other activities.

- Don't go to bed until you're sleepy.

- Don't have screen time for an hour before you go to bed.

DISCOLORED SKIN, FINGERNAILS, AND TOENAILS

If you have radiation, your skin may become discolored. Some creams may help; ask your radiation nurse for suggestions. In any case, the discoloration will disappear by itself sooner or later.

I wish I could tell you why some treatments cause fingernails and toenails to darken and get ridges, but nobody seems to be able to tell me the reason. If it does happen to you, though, don't worry. It's yet another side effect of meds. The experts tell you to keep your nails clean and dry and not to wear fake nails. It's okay, though, to use nail polish. Consider using cold therapy gloves during treatments to reduce side effects.

DIMINISHED LIBIDO

This is a natural result of treatment. Don't worry; it'll come back.

VAGINAL DRYNESS

Vaginal dryness occurs when menopause kicks in because of the discontinuation of estrogen production. Estrogen helps keep the vagina elastic and lubricated. Use water-based lubricants such as K-Y Jelly, not oil-based lubricants such as Vaseline, to ease the discomfort.

YOUR WEIGHT: GOOD NEWS AND BAD NEWS

Ask your doctor if you should expect weight loss or weight gain. In either case, it's best not to be surprised.

The good news: If you've wished you could get those last few pounds off, a slimmer, trimmer you may well be in sight. Sixty percent of people in cancer treatment lose weight.

Granted, there are far less extreme ways to reduce weight. But for me, the thought of *any* benefits from having this crummy disease was a ray of light. The prospect of losing weight wasn't just a ray; it was a three-hundred-watt bulb.

By the way, this definitely is not the time to *try* to lose weight if you're not gaining weight.

The bad news: If you've wished and wished you could lose those last few pounds, hope that you aren't in the other 40 percent who maintain or gain weight during treatment. Much to my chagrin, I found myself in that 40 percent. I was devastated. As if losing all my hair wasn't bad enough, I was also watching the scale move in the wrong direction, and I'd had no idea that was even a possibility. I thought everybody who was in treatment lost weight. When I finally mentioned to my oncology nurse that I'd gained fifteen pounds—I'd wondered why he couldn't tell; everybody else could!—he casually assured me that "the chemo is causing that." I could have used that info a lot earlier!

Why do some people gain weight during treatment, while others lose it? Some chemotherapies, medications—particularly steroids—hormone regimens, and the onset of treatment-induced menopause all trigger weight gain. In my case, the particular chemo I was being treated with was a factor. Apparently it had increased my appetite—believe it or not, I hadn't noticed—and since I'd expected to lose weight, and was also feeling sorry for myself, I ate whatever I pleased. Who knew that my new status of cancer patient hadn't made me immune to weight gain? To add insult to injury, since the chemo had thrown me into early meno-pause, my metabolism had plummeted. Needless to say, I was not amused.

According to the American Cancer Society, steroids in particular can cause extreme hunger and cravings. Knowing this in advance can help you curb your eating when you want to eat.

Water retention is also a common cause of weight gain, so reducing the amount of salt in your diet may help you keep the extra pounds off as well. It's a good idea to stay as active as possible and exercise regularly, as long as your doctor says it's okay. Even if you simply walk around the house, you're burning calories.

MANAGING PAIN

I've developed a new philosophy . . .
I only dread one day at a time.
—Charles Schulz

The best way to control pain is to get it treated early. The sooner you ask for help, the easier it will be to alleviate it. Don't hold off as long as you can without taking pain medicine. The only thing that suffering with pain achieves is that it forces your body to use your energy to fight pain instead of using it to fight cancer.

There are many safe, effective pain medications available today, and the more feedback you can give your doctor about what you're experiencing, the sooner you'll find relief.

Don't wait for your doctor to ask whether you're experiencing pain. Tell him. Pain management is a very important part of cancer treatment, and experts say that with the rarest exceptions, nobody with cancer should be in pain for long periods of time.

> The only thing that suffering with pain achieves is that it forces your body to use your energy to fight pain instead of using it to fight cancer.

Keep a pain journal. On a scale of one to ten—least to most pain—note how much or little pain you've experienced during the day. You can also track when and where pain occurs, how long it lasts, and the side effects you're experiencing from your pain medicine.

Nondrug treatments for pain include relaxation and breathing exercises, massage, biofeedback, imagery, acupuncture, distraction, skin stimulation, pressure, and vibration. The American Cancer Society offers extremely helpful instructions for things you can do yourself to deal with pain. See www.cancer.org, the section entitled "Pain Control: A Guide for People with Cancer and Their Families."

> **Most important:** Don't be a martyr! There are no prizes for suffering in silence.

Most important: Don't be a martyr! There are no prizes for suffering in silence.

4

Your Mind and Spirit

Between stimulus and response there is a space.
In that space is our power to choose our response.
In our response lies our growth and our freedom.

—Viktor Frankl

Remember: You Come First

This is the time to take care of your needs and put them first—no matter who else you're caring for. Besides, if your own needs aren't being met, you can't take care of others—whether or not you have cancer.

Right now, taking care of yourself means saying to visitors, "I really appreciate your visit. I'm a little tired now, but I'd love to visit when I have a little more energy."

It's okay to cry. Just don't get too used to it.

Right now, taking care of yourself means saying to visitors, "I really appreciate your visit. I'm a little tired now, but I'd love to visit when I have a little more energy." Taking care of yourself means telling people what you really could use help with when they ask what they can do for you.

Stiff upper lips aren't all they're cracked up to be. It's okay to have a "sad day." It's okay to cry. Just don't get too used to it.

How Do You Know How You're Coping with Cancer When You've Never Had It Before?

It only began to hit me that I really had cancer after the tornado of phone calls, diagnoses, appointments, arrangements, surgery, and everything else began to die down. Adrenaline is a wonderful thing. It puts us in high gear and turns us into temporary superheroes. But after the alarms and sirens fade, so does our adrenaline supply.

After the early days of crisis, I began to realize that I hadn't just completed a limited engagement starring in *Michelle Gets Cancer* and was now back to my real life.

Cancer *was my* real life. People would ask, "How are you coping?" and I realized I didn't know. I'd never done it before.

The American Cancer Society website (cancer.org) offers great help with coping. Here are some highlights:

- Stay as active as you can.

- Eat balanced meals.

- Don't try to do everything yourself.

- Talk about your feelings, no matter what they are. If you're uncomfortable talking with a friend or loved one, don't hesitate to get help. A therapist can be invaluable at a time like this.

- Check out Cancer Survivors Network (csn.cancer.org). It provides chat boards categorized by cancer type where you can ask questions and learn from others who are dealing with the same issues you are.

Remember: You're in a temporary phase right now called the new normal. Be patient with yourself. Cut yourself a lot of slack. Don't lose hope. Don't lose your sense of humor.

Be patient with yourself. Cut yourself a lot of slack. Don't lose hope. Don't lose your sense of humor.

It's okay to cry. Did you know tears release toxins? Just don't get too used to it.

Your Mind: You're Not Losing It—You Just Have Chemo Brain

Not too long into my chemotherapy, I began to realize that my memory was fading fast. I was already worried sick about my poor body. Now I was getting worried about my mind too. I couldn't concentrate; I'd forget conversations I'd had just hours ago; I'd be sure I'd finished a task only to find it later partially undone. It wasn't until a year after I had finished my treatment that my sister called to tell me she'd read about something called chemo brain. Chemo brain—slang for *cognitive deficits*—is an unfortunate possible side effect of all cancer treatments, although not everyone experiences it. It isn't yet known why some people get it and others don't. Chemo brain symptoms include:

- Short-term memory loss

- Difficulty concentrating / shortened attention span

- Difficulty retrieving words

- Difficulty organizing and planning

According to Dr. Christina A. Meyers, former chief of neuropsychology at M. D. Anderson Cancer Center, one of the best things you can do to reduce the severity of your symptoms is to introduce your brain to entirely new, different activities than it's used to. For example:

- Do crossword puzzle or sudoku.

- Learn to do needlepoint or take a stab at knitting.

- Listen to different kinds of music and read different kinds of books than you usually do. If you're a mystery fan, read a biography. If you love Frank Sinatra, see if jazz strikes your fancy—or maybe you're a country music fan, and you just don't know it!

- Try anything you haven't done before that will surprise your brain; it will be helpful.

- Listen to relaxation background music, guided meditation, and visualization exercises.

- Ask your doctor if you're a candidate for Ritalin to help alleviate poor concentration as well as fatigue.

Chemo brain will eventually go away, but it usually lasts for up to a year after chemo ends. No one knows what specifically causes it, but I, for one, am grateful just to know that my scary mental lapses were artificially induced, and I have a good chance of . . . what was I saying?

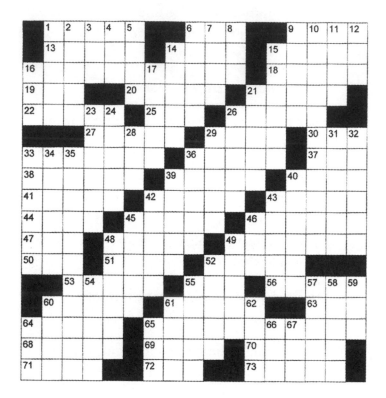

ACROSS

1 Whole ball of wax

6 Forty winks

9 Cries on cue

13 Rotund

14 Blown away

15 Windy City airport

16 A day with hair

18 Sports event site

19 ___ de-France (region ringing Paris)

20 Show contempt

21 ___ on earth

22 Self-important ones

25 ___ capita

26 Cape _____ (Africa's westernmost point)

27 "Be prepared" is his motto

29 We all want to do it

30 Blushing

33 ___ group

36 Ornate

37 Jalopy

38 French star

39 It goes with hope and charity

40 Speedy sled

41 Dragged behind

42 Muddies the waters

43 Chorines

44 Unlatches, to poets

45 Teems

46 Zellweger and Adoree

47 City in Iran

48 Tom Sawyer's aunt

49 It's "the best policy"

50 ___ Paulo, Brazil

51 Feels remorse

52 Military cabal

53 Motorists' mishaps

55 ___ up the works (thwart)

56 Bridge triumphs

60 Light carriages

61 It's usually given in a parlor

63 Sticky stuff

64 Liquor, slangily

65 Winston Churchill said it

68 Kind of crust

69 Rathskeller quaffs

70 Cuts of pork

71 Molt

72 Alcove

73 Maternally related

DOWN

1 Hammers, wrenches, and saws

2 Bassoons' kin

3 Turner or Danson

4 ___ Wednesday

5 Pastures

6 US consumer activist

7 Culture medium

8 Fork over

9 In the lead

10 The best things since sliced bread

11 Accurate

12 Match a poker bet

14 Hail; welcome

15 With excessiveness

16 Actress Scala

17 Computer data entered

21 Pinkish-yellow hue

23 Catches sight of

24 Rebuke

26 Air ducts

28 Argentite is one

29 Showers heavy sleet

31 Small seabird

32 Formal attire

33 First US saint, et al.

34 Idealized spot

35 Never underestimate it

36 Pixie

39 Diamond goofs

40 Hereditary

42 Parts in a play

43 Blokes

45 Gets sulky

46 Director Howard

48 Petition to God

49 You need it to get through cancer

52 Burlap fibers

54 Lolled, lounged

55 Judge's mallet

57 Celeb's representative

58 Mickey or Minnie

59 Drench

60 Next year's jr.

61 Give an account of

62 Make eyes at

64 City conveyance

65 Glasgow veto

66 Particle

67 By way of

Dealing with Depression

It's one thing to be sad. If you weren't sad about having cancer, that would be very strange. But there's a real difference between being sad and being depressed. At any given time, 10 percent of the American population suffers from depression. Thirty percent of cancer patients suffer from it, so if you think you might be depressed, the odds are that you are.

I've suffered from bouts of major depression in my life, and I can assure you that you really don't want to be in the middle of cancer and depression at the same time. One is bad enough, but in combination, they're brutal.

ONGOING SYMPTOMS OF DEPRESSION

Symptoms of depression include:

- Frequent feelings of hopelessness, despair, and inadequacy

- Little, if any, interest in things that used to be pleasurable

- Crying often and easily

- Thoughts of suicide

- Loss of interest in sex

- Extreme feelings of worthlessness and guilt

If you experience some or all of these feelings much or most of the time, please, please tell your medical team as soon as you realize that they're not going away. Your body needs all of its energy to heal. Why force it to undergo the added stress of depression? Also, the medical community has determined there is a strong connection between depression and a suppressed immune system, and you especially need your immune system to work as well as possible right now. So if you're depressed, please get help.

Finally, don't refuse to take an antidepressant if it's recommended. I know how hard it is to accept the fact that you might need them. But I can tell you from experience that taking them is like taking aspirin or allergy medicine. In fact, if you've ever taken Zyban to quit smoking, then you've already taken an antidepressant. Zyban is actually Wellbutrin, one of the most widely used antidepressants in the country.

Remember, don't suffer in silence. Don't just hope the depression will go away by itself. It won't. Tell your doctor as soon as you think that you might be depressed. Consider seeing a therapist.

Like pain, the earlier depression is treated, the more quickly and easily it will be alleviated. Not to mention that you'll avoid unnecessary strain on your already overworked body.

Matters of the Spirit

*Faith is taking the first step even when
you don't see the whole staircase.*

—Martin Luther King Jr.

Whatever your beliefs are—or aren't—it's just as important to nourish your soul as it is to feed your body. For whatever reason, it's often when we're in crisis that we begin to explore things of the spirit, whether by prayer, meditation, listening to Bach or Mozart, or simply being quiet with our eyes closed.

The National Institute of Mental Health has determined that people with cancer often have less anxiety, depression, and even pain when they feel strong spiritual connections. Many studies have shown conclusively that prayerful consciousness has been shown to inhibit the growth of cancer cells, increase the supply of oxygen to the blood, protect red blood cells, and alter blood chemistry. Some studies have even shown that prayer on behalf of a sick person has some positive effect on the healing process.

Prayer has always been an important part of my life. But after I was diagnosed, it became even more so. Not only did I find myself praying more intensely and mindfully than before but also wanted to be prayed *for*. In fact, when people wanted to know what they could do for me, I found myself asking them to pray—not only for me but also for my husband and family and my medical team. That was the gift I wanted most. Trust me, I'm pretty materialistic, so no one was more surprised at this desire for prayer than me.

Most of the time, my own prayers consisted of my just talking to God . . . not out loud—the last thing I needed was to be given a psychiatric diagnosis. Much of the time, I was pretty mad at God for letting this happen to me. I hadn't married until I was forty-five, and I'd been married for only two years. What if I didn't make it? So I'd rail at him. *"What were you thinking?"* I'd ask. I figured that if

God is God, then he can take my yelling at him. But I also asked for peace and strength and comfort—and healing, of course. During the process, I became less angry and more peaceful.

I know I said earlier that when you have cancer, you need to put yourself first and that it's all about you. Well, I largely believe that, particularly if you're a *pleaser*, as I am. But that isn't entirely true. Yes, your first priority right now is to handle your cancer as best you can. That means saying no to well-intentioned people who mean to help but actually are taking up more of your energy than you can spare. It means resting when you feel you should be doing the dishes. But here's what it doesn't mean. It doesn't mean that you shouldn't think of others.

In my experience, prayer is richer when it includes praying for others' needs as well as my own. There's no shortage of suffering and need in our world, and nothing is off limits in my prayer.

One day while I was in the hospital, I got a new roommate. She was distressed because she'd lost her eye drops. She was making frantic calls to friends and family and shouting at every nurse and orderly that she needed them to look for her drops. She was nearly hysterical and very angry. And she was in a bed about three feet from me. I was not happy.

Later that afternoon, a chaplain walked in and greeted her. She wasn't warm and wonderful, but that didn't deter him. After a little bit of talk, he asked her if she wanted him to pray for her. I expected her to turn him down outright, but she accepted his offer. As he prayed, and I listened from behind the curtain, I felt noticeably calmer—and he wasn't even praying for me! I decided that maybe I should include her in my own prayers. As I silently prayed, I found myself praying for all the patients on that cancer floor and for those who attended them. Since that experience, I've learned that there are many reasons to pray for others even when I'm suffering. Praying for others expands one's sense of compassion. It's also often a reminder that while my own situation is very serious, I'm not the only one suffering. That reminder helps provide a sense of perspective for me. I realize that even in my own depth of problems, I'm not alone. And yes, there are others who are in even more dire straits. I've come to believe that just as doing a kindness for someone else feeds something in me, so does praying.

Prayers for Healing and Peace

Here are several prayers from a variety of faiths that you may find helpful. Each denomination is represented by a prayer that was written by a member of the clergy who is no stranger to cancer.

CATHOLIC

Peregrine, the Patron Saint of Cancer

Peregrine Laziosi was born in 1260 in Forli, Italy, to a very wealthy family. His youth was spent selfishly and was monopolized by material possessions. He found his way into politics and became very anti-Catholic. Peregrine converted, however, after beating Philip Benizi, a future saint, and seeing the holy man turn the cheek and pray for his attacker. Peregrine later joined the Servite Order and spent many years in solitude. The gentle confessor fell victim to a horrific cancer of his foot that spread rapidly. While awaiting amputation, Peregrine spent the night before the operation in prayer and received a vision of Jesus healing his malady instantly. By the next morning, his foot was completely cured.

Prayer to St. Peregrine

> *O great Peregrine,*
> *I am inspired by your faith, bravery and stamina.*
> *Pray that I can be as strong and prayerful as you were.*
> *Ask God to get me through this painful experience*
> *   with dignity and laughter.*
> *Pray for* my *supportive family and my loving friends,*
> *   as God sees me through to a total recovery.*
> *Amen.*

—from *Saintly Advice*

PROTESTANT

Eternal and loving God, in the midst of illness I will
*   praise your holy name.*
Even as I fight this fateful disease, I will affirm that
*   life is good and a blessing to be savored.*

By your grace, help me find something amazing to
cherish and thank you for every day, something,
perhaps, that I might not have noticed when I
was well.
Firm me in my determination not to allow
cancer to rob me of my values or my personality,
or alienate me from those I love, including you,
O Lord.
Precious Father, get me through the hard days.
Hold my hand and do not let fear conquer me.
Above all, open me to your healing power, for I pray
to you through your Son, Jesus Christ.
Amen.

—Rev. Dr. Noel Vanek, Pastor, Community Church of the
Pelhams, Pelham, New York

JEWISH

May the One who blessed our Patriarchs Abraham,
Isaac and Jacob and our Matriarchs Sarah,
Rebecca, Rachel, and Leah bless me in my jour-
ney seeking a Refuah Shleimah, a healing of Body
and Spirit.
Please bless my clinicians not only in treating my
illness,
but also in supporting me as a unique spirit created
in Your Image.
Please bless my family and friends as they support me.

*May I be blessed to feel Your love through them. May
they be strengthened in Your love as well.*
*Please allow me to feel Your Presence in the moun-
tains and valleys—for I know that wherever I go,
You shall be there.*
*Help me to accept and love who I am in the moment—
emotionally, physically and spiritually—as I
know that You, my Creator who knew me in the
womb, accept and love me.*
*May I be restored to a healing of soul and
body.*

—Rabbi Nathan Goldberg

ISLAMIC

*With G-D's name the merciful benefactor, the merci-
ful Redeemer,*
*Dear G-D, please give us what is good in this life,
and what is good in the next life, and save us,
because nothing can save us except you.*
We humbly ask you to heal us, very soon.
*Please make this process easy for us and do not
place a burden on us greater than we can
bear.*
*We also ask that you bless our families, because we
don't know why we are tested with so much
illness and hardships in our lives.*

Please give them the strength, the courage and the
faith to deal with anything that comes in the
future.
Bless the doctors and nurses who care for us, that they
make right decisions.
Now we ask you to bless the sick and infirm, espe-
cially the children, wherever they may be on this
earth, because after all the earth is our home.
Above all, please bless us to be well and continue to
live a long, good and healthy life, if it pleases you.
Amen.

—Imam Yusuf Hasan, BCC, Chaplain, Memorial
Sloan Kettering Cancer Center

Encouragement, Comfort, and Strength from the Bible

I read some books while I was in treatment that encouraged me and gave me new insights into the spiritual aspects of going through cancer, some specific to the disease and others more general. But the most encouraging, comforting ones for me that gave me injections of peace and strength were from the Bible. I've included some passages from a few of them here that were among the most helpful to me:

But now the Lord who created you, O Israel, says: Do not be afraid, for I have ransomed you; I have called you by name;

you are mine. When you go through deep waters and great trouble, I will be with you. When you go through rivers of difficulty, you will not drown! When you walk through the fire of oppression, you will not be burned up—the flames will not consume you. (Isa 43:1–2, The Living Bible)

I look to the hills! Where will I find help? It will come from the LORD, who created the heavens and the earth. (Ps 121:1–2, CEV)

Even though I walk through the valley of the shadow of death, I will fear no evil, for you are with me. (Ps 23:4, NIV)

Do not fear, I will help you. (Isa 41:13, NIV)

The LORD bless you and keep you; the LORD make his face to shine upon you and be gracious to you; the LORD turn his face toward you and give you peace. (Num 6:24–26, NIV)

Be strong and courageous. Do not be terrified; do not be discouraged, for the LORD your God will be with you wherever you go. (Josh 1:9, NIV)

He rescues and he saves; he performs signs and wonders in the heavens and on the earth. He has rescued Daniel from the power of the lions. (Dan 6:27, NIV)

BIBLE PASSAGES TO COMFORT AND ENCOURAGE

For I know the plans I have for you," declares the LORD, "plans to prosper you and not to harm you, plans to give you a hope and a future. (Jer 29:11)

I lift up my eyes to the hills—where does my help come from? My help comes from the LORD, the Maker of heaven and earth. He will not let your foot slip—he who watches over you will not slumber; indeed, he who watches over Israel will neither slumber nor sleep. The LORD watches over you—the LORD is your shade at your right hand; the sun will not harm you by day, nor the moon by night. The LORD will keep you from all harm—he will watch over your life; the LORD will watch over your coming and going both now and forevermore. (Ps 121)

But those who hope in the LORD will renew their strength. They will soar on wings like eagles; they will run and not grow weary, and they will walk, and not be faint. (Isa 40:31)

The LORD is my shepherd; I shall not be in want. He makes me lie down in green pastures, he leads me beside quiet waters, he restores my soul. He guides me in the paths of righteousness for his name's sake. Even though I walk through the valley of the shadow of death, I will fear no

evil, for you are with me; your rod and your staff, they com-
fort me. You prepare a table before me in the presence of my
enemies. You anoint my head with oil; my cup overflows.
Surely goodness and love will follow me all the days of my
life, and I will dwell in the house of the LORD forever.
(Ps 23)

I have told you these things, so that in me you may have
peace. In this world you will have trouble. But take heart!
I have overcome the world. (John 16:33)

Are not two sparrows sold for a penny? Yet not one of them
will fall to the ground apart from the will of your Father.
And even the very hairs of your head are all numbered. So
don't be afraid; you are worth more than many sparrows.
(Matt 10:29–31)

He who dwells in the shelter of the Most High will rest in
the shadow of the Almighty. I will say of the LORD, "He
is my refuge and my fortress, my God, in whom I trust."
Surely he will save you from the fowler's snare and from
the deadly pestilence. He will cover you with his feathers,
and under his wings you will find refuge; his faithfulness
will be your shield and rampart. You will not fear the
terror of night, nor the arrow that flies by day, nor the
pestilence that stalks in the darkness, nor the plague that
destroys at midday. A thousand may fall at your side, ten
thousand at your right hand, but it will not come near you.
(Ps 91:1–7)

Cast all your anxiety on him because he cares for you.
(I Pet 5:7)

Come to me, all you who are weary and burdened, and I will give you rest. Take my yoke upon you and learn from me, for I am gentle and humble in heart, and you will find rest for your souls. For my yoke is easy and my burden is light. (Matt 11:28–30)

And when Daniel was lifted from the [lions'] den, no wound was found on him, because he had trusted in his God. (Dan 6:23)

Maintaining a Positive Attitude without Feeling Like a Human Smiley Face

THE HOUSE OF A THOUSAND MIRRORS

Long ago in a tiny village, there was a place called the House of a Thousand Mirrors. A little dog decided to visit the house. He was an unhappy dog, and his natural expression was a cross between a scowl and a sneer. As he entered the large house, he saw a thousand mean- and scary-looking dogs staring back at him. He immediately backed away and let out a low growl to protect himself, and just as he did, all one thousand of the mean dogs growled back at him. Of course, he ran out of the house immediately and thought, *What a terrible place that is. I'll never go back there again.*

Not long afterward, another dog decided to visit the house. As he approached, he saw how beautiful and inviting it looked and couldn't wait to go inside. He smiled and wagged his tail in anticipation of his adventure. As he pushed open the door, he was greeted by a thousand dogs with wagging tails and big smiles approaching him. Of course, he was thrilled; he had a thousand new friends he was sure would become his lifelong buddies.

The moral of this folktale is that the world gives back to us what we give out to the world. That's not to say we should pretend that everything's great when in fact we're going through one of the hardest challenges of our lives. But it *is* true that the more positive you can be right now, the more smiling puppies you'll have to cheer you on.

Helpful Self-Talk

Often, in an effort to make you feel better, people will say some pretty annoying things; *infuriating* is probably a more accurate term. Having cancer is *not* a blessing in disguise. The fact that you don't have a worse cancer is not terribly comforting. As wonderful as it is to learn how many people love and care about you, there are other ways to learn that same thing that aren't nearly as dangerous, devastating, or life-altering as having cancer.

But there are some things that are true and can bring comfort and a new perspective on this crummy situation. These are some that have been of help to me:

A year from today this will be behind me.
A year from today, I'll have hair!

My lack of hair means that the chemo is working.
I am not *a statistic.*
I am the CEO of my health. I have control over
many things, and this is the time for me to
take hold of and maintain and use that power.

There are more people who care deeply and want to support me now than perhaps at any time in my life. I need to accept their generosity, and one day I will reciprocate. If they sometimes say dumb things, it's because they're frightened on my behalf. I need to give them the benefit of the doubt and accept with grace their stabs at comforting me.

Cancer is not a death sentence. In fact, more people die of heart disease every year than of cancer. Yet we don't view people with heart disease as living under the specter of death. Just because an idea is commonly believed, that doesn't make it true.

Just because your prognosis is better than mine doesn't mean you'll outlive me. Granted, this is a little hard-nosed, and it's probably better if you don't go around saying it to people. But the truth is nobody knows what will happen next week, or tomorrow, or in an hour.

Cancer sucks. There are pins, T-shirts, and baseball caps that say "Cancer Sucks." It's short and to the point and, in my opinion, sums up the situation to a T. For some mysterious reason, it made me feel better just to say those two little words every now and then.

I'm going to make cancer history. Get it? Make cancer *history.*

Just because I'm not cured yet, it doesn't mean that I can't experience healing. As you know, there isn't a lot about cancer that could be called *beneficial.* But like many other hard experiences in life, even this terrible journey can be—in fact, often is—a catalyst for healing in areas that will serve us well both in the short term and the long run. Chances are you've already experienced an outpouring of care and kindness from others whom you wouldn't have expected to be so giving. Cancer causes us to reexamine our priorities and often triggers new, healthier decisions about where we will spend our energy and emotions.

STUCK ON PLANET CANCER, OR WOULD IT HELP TO SEE A COUNSELOR?

I mentioned that when I was diagnosed, I felt as if my body had betrayed me. In fact, my body suddenly seemed like another entity—part of me yet at the same time separate. "Who are you? How could you do this?" I'd ask it. "We've been together for forty-seven years. I thought I knew you. I thought you liked me!" I felt alone in a way that I could hardly describe. I was in uncharted territory—Planet Cancer, I called it—and as much as others loved and supported me, they couldn't be there with me.

On Earth, I knew how to navigate through my life pretty well. But on Planet Cancer, I was constantly tripping over one new fear or another: physical fears, the fear of being a burden, concerns about how my family would be affected by my illness, financial concerns, not to mention some anger and resentment.

Being a big believer in not reinventing the wheel, I decided that if there were ways to handle having cancer that had already been devised, then I'd rather not try to come up with them myself.

In therapy, I learned new ways to deal with many of my fears and upsets that have served me well long after my illness passed. I also learned that, unlike most any other place, you never need to censor yourself in a therapist's office in order to protect other people or to hide reactions that you think are "unacceptable." And if you're fortunate enough to find a therapist as extraordinary as mine, then you may well find that it's the one doctor's appointment that you actually look forward to.

One of my mantras over the course of my treatment was "Whatever it takes, do it." In other words, this isn't the time to be practical. Whatever it takes to feel better, if it's feasible, legal, and you can afford it, do it. And I did. And it helped.

TRIED AND TRUE WAYS TO MAKE THINGS A LITTLE BETTER

- Treat yourself to something special after each treatment—assuming you'll feel like it—and decide on it in advance. Have tea with a friend, go out for ice cream with another friend, or pick up a magazine that you usually don't buy.

- Keep a cache of fizzling bath salts; beautiful candles; a CD player; and a brand-new fluffy, soft towel in the bathroom and lock yourself in for a relaxing home spa treatment. T. J. Maxx and Marshalls have indulgent bath products at a discount.

- Discover the wonderful world of home shopping networks, where you can find things that you didn't even know existed and now can't live without. Truly, they became some of my favorite destinations, and I never got my Christmas shopping done faster or more successfully.

- Plan something special. It's important to make plans, for both the short term and long term. Imaging and visualization are important tools for promoting health, and that includes visualizing and anticipating special events, both large and small—things like a cruise, a few days at a spa, a splurge at your favorite store, a trip to a foreign country, or a trip to Bath and Body Works.

I decided that I wanted to take a fancy cruise with my husband along the Mediterranean coast to celebrate the return of my hair. I spent countless hours researching the possibilities and finally came up with the perfect trip. I got so much satisfaction and pleasure from planning it that when we ended up canceling, for unrelated reasons, I hardly felt deprived: it almost seemed to me as if I'd taken it!

The Value of Journaling

Apart from counseling, writing in my journal was the most helpful way of uncovering, sorting through, and examining all the stuff that was dropping into my life like asteroids on Planet Cancer. Like counseling, my journal was a safe place to express everything I was feeling, and I often found that the very process of writing clarified why I was worried about a particular thing or how I'd handle a situation the next time it arose.

Studies at major institutions around the country, including Ohio State University, Southern Methodist University, and M. D. Anderson Cancer Center, have determined that the practice of writing provides the following overall health benefits: pain reduction, immune function improvement—including an increase in T cell counts—resistance to minor illnesses such as colds and the flu, and lower blood pressure and heart rate. The connections between writing and increased physical well-being are so interesting to the medical community that the National Institutes of Health is sponsoring a five-year study to examine the physical and psychological benefits of counseling and journaling in cancer patients.

GETTING STARTED

Buy an inexpensive notebook to write in. Don't buy a fancy blank book. Spiral is an easier format for writing; more important, fancy books can be very intimidating and become obstacles to writing. If typing is easier; keep your journal on your computer. This is not for an audience or for publication. This is for your eyes and your use. You might never want to share it, and that's fine. Consider the following:

- If anybody else uses your computer, consider using a boring alias for the file, such as "Physics" or "Cleaning Supplies." Nobody will be tempted to peek!

- Because starting a journal can be daunting, give yourself permission to write for just five minutes. You can do anything for five minutes. If you want to stop then, no problem. Chances are, though, that once you start writing, the time will fly.

- If you haven't kept a journal before, it may be a little intimidating to start. After you get the hang of it, you won't have to think about what you're going to write about. For now, here are a couple of suggestions just to get you going. First, you've been through an awful lot in a short time. What's happened up until now? How did you learn about your diagnosis? How have you been surprised by how people have responded to the news? What treatment(s) are you having? How are you getting along with your medical team? How do you feel about what's happened to you? Remember, be honest. This journal is for your eyes only.

Keeping a journal serves a number of purposes: it's the chronicle of a time in your life like no other. Hard as it is to believe, the time will come when you don't remember as much of this marathon as you expect to now.

Perhaps most important, this inanimate object that probably cost only a few dollars will gradually become your confidant. You'll be able to tell it things that you may not tell anyone else. By telling those things, you'll probably gain insights and even some answers to some very thorny issues. Silly as it may sound, your journal will become an intimate friend.

Handling the Holidays

The bottom line for handling the holiday season is: do—or don't do—whatever you need to in order to get through it. That might mean sleeping through it if you don't have little ones or pets. There aren't any good one-size-fits-all answers to the holiday issue, but here are a few tactics that can help a bit:

- Accept an invitation or two if you're up to it. It really is better to be with other people than to be sitting alone in your living room. Don't feel obligated to accept all invitations—or even most. Just don't be a hermit.

- Take a vacation from the busy work associated with holidays. This is the year that you can get away with anything, so do what you want to do and forget the rest. It'll all be there for you to do next year. If you don't want to send out cards, don't.

- If you do want to send out holiday cards, donate to a charity that will send out holiday cards to your list, with a note in each card indicating that you've made a donation in the person's name. Then you'll have taken care of cards and gifts. This can get expensive, so be choosy.

- If you're buying gifts, find something that most anyone would like—a little flashlight, a purse pen—and then buy ten or twenty of them. Give them to everyone on your list within reason.

- By now, you know for sure that it isn't presents or parties or fattening foods that give the holidays their meaning, so don't feel pressured to do anything except be with the people you love—on your terms, of course.

Important Documents for Peace of Mind

All adults, regardless of their state of health, should take steps to let others know exactly what kind of medical treatment they want—or don't want—in case they're unable to communicate their own wishes due to an accident or illness. It's even more important for you to do this, not because you expect to die any time soon but because it's the kind of thing that needs to be in place well before you need it.

According to the American Bar Association (ABA), even though every state has its own rules governing the documents below, health-care providers generally will honor your wishes regardless of which form you use or where you drew it up. The ABA does recommend, though, that if you spend significant amounts of time in another state, you secure these documents there as well as at your primary residence.

The following is a list of documents you need in order to guarantee that your wishes will be followed if your ability to make decisions is ever compromised. They can all be rescinded or changed at any time.

APPOINTMENT OF HEALTH-CARE PROXY (ALSO KNOWN AS DURABLE POWER OF ATTORNEY)

This is a legal document through which you appoint someone who, in most states, must be at least eighteen years old to make decisions about your care if you are unable to make them. That person has broad authority over your care and has access to all of your medical records. It is recommended that you name one person to serve at a time and that you choose at least one backup person.

LIVING WILL

This legal document allows you to specify your preferences regarding your treatment and care if you become terminally ill or if it is not expected that you will recover from physical or mental disability or disease. The will can give general guidelines, such as requesting no life support if you are terminally ill. It can also include specific instructions regarding feeding-tube use or the use of a respirator or cardiopulmonary resuscitation, for example. A living will can be changed or canceled at any time. For more information, go to the US Living Will Registry website (uslivingwillregistry.com).

RELEASE OF MEDICAL INFORMATION

If you want anybody besides your first-degree relative to have access to any medical information concerning your condition, then it's imperative that you secure one of these releases for each person you want to keep in the loop. Like all of the documents listed here, this can be rescinded or changed at any time. But if you don't have it in place and you become unable to express your own wishes, then no exceptions will be made.

5

Humor

It Really Is the Best Medicine (Well, at Least It Doesn't Make You Nauseous)

Laughter makes the unbearable bearable, and a patient with a well-developed sense of humor has a better chance of recovery than an individual who seldom laughs.
—Dr. Bernie Siegel

To succeed in life, you need three things: a wishbone, a backbone, and a funny bone.
—Reba McEntire

What's Funny about Cancer?

That's easy. The answer is *nothing*. There's nothing even mildly amusing about cancer, much less funny. But there are books, scientific studies from prestigious universities, and powerful first-person accounts that attest to the healing power of humor. Not curing power but healing power.

When you laugh, your chest, abdominal muscles, diaphragm, and lungs contract, giving your body the equivalent of a mini workout. Your heart rate and blood pressure increase as if you were doing aerobic exercise. Adrenaline is pumped into your blood, and endorphins are released.

Medical science has found that endorphins trigger runner's high, a sort of euphoria, and help strengthen the immune system. It's also established that laughter increases antibodies, activates T immune cells, and decreases stress hormones and that laughter helps to decrease pain by causing physical relaxation and reducing anxiety.

In the movie *Patch Adams*, based on a true story, Robin Williams plays a young physician whose extraordinary use of fun, humor, and laughter transforms the attitudes of seriously ill patients of all ages. If you haven't seen it, do.

Some hospitals are introducing "humor rooms" in their oncology wings, which include players for comedy DVDs, games, toys, costumes, NERF balls, and bubbles. And they're on the adult floors.

So even though there's nothing funny about having cancer, there are reasons to see the humor in life, even some of the ironic, outrageous situations that arise from being in this awful situation. Don't forgo any opportunity to laugh that comes along.

Jokes Only a Cancer Patient Could Love

A doctor tells his patient, "The tests show your cancer is advanced. You have six months to live." "But, Doctor, I can't pay off my medical bills in six months," the patient exclaims. "In that case," says the doctor, "you have a year."

A doctor finally reaches her patient after several days of phone tag to report the results of his medical tests. "Do you want the good news or the bad news?" she asks. "The good news," the patient replies. "You have forty-eight hours to live," says the doctor. "That's the good news?" cries the patient. "What could possibly be the bad news?" "I called last week."

Paul and Jack, two old baseball buddies, both with cancer, are chatting on a park bench. "I hope they have a baseball team in heaven," says the first. "Me too," his friend replies. "Tell you what: If I die first, I'll give you a message about whether there's baseball in heaven. If you die first, you can do the same for me," he suggests. A year later, Paul is dead, and Jack is on the park bench. He hears, "Jack, it's me, Paul. I have great news! There really is a baseball team in heaven." "Thank God," Jack says, "now I can die in peace." "I'm glad you feel that way," Paul says, "because you're pitching tomorrow."

A very religious woman is diagnosed with cancer. Certain that God will heal her, she turns down treatment from a cancer surgeon, a radiologist, and an oncologist. She soon dies, and the first thing she says to God is "I believed in you. I thought you were going to heal me. What happened?" "Got me," says God. "I sent you a surgeon, a radiologist, and an oncologist!"

SIX WAYS YOU KNOW YOUR DOCTOR IS AN ONCOLOGIST

He asks you if you want to have a port, and he's not offering you a drink.

Even though he is wearing a white lab coat and not a military uniform, he keeps using words like *battle*, *fight*, and *destroy*.

He tries to explain to you why a low grade on your report is better than a high grade.

He talks a lot about trials, and as far as you know, he's not a lawyer or a judge.

He explains your treatment series, and you keep wondering where the facial and massage part comes in.

He tells you that you are on a protocol, and it doesn't seem to fit with the dictionary definition: a form of ceremony and etiquette observed by diplomats and heads of state.

POSITIVE THINGS ABOUT NOT HAVING HAIR—NOT A HUGE LIST

The shower and sink drains have stopped getting clogged.

You now prefer hair-raising movies.

You can remove your hair when you weigh yourself.

People can see a strong resemblance between you and your new grandchild.

You don't have to wash your hair.

You don't have to shave your legs or your chin.

You don't have to worry about your bikini line.

If you go to the bowling alley and there's a long wait for a lane, just put your turban on, place your bowling ball in front of you, and charge for fortune readings.

6

Well-Meaning Family, Friends, and Strangers

Your Spouse

Not to engage in one-upmanship, but did I mention that shortly after I went into remission, my husband learned that he had prostate cancer? Until then, I'd considered myself the cancer expert in residence. But my experience as his caregiver showed me a side of cancer I hadn't expected. For example, what could be worse than being nauseous, bald, bandaged, green, in pain, and exhausted? I'm not sure. But watching someone you love be nauseous, bald, bandaged, green, in pain, and exhausted—and not being able to do anything about it—is right up there.

Here are a few things that you and your partner can do for each other that will help bring you through this closer than you were before:

- Remember that he's feeling as frightened, besieged, and overwhelmed as you are. Even though you need him to be strong, cut him some slack. You've both been hit by a two-ton truck.

- Stay in touch with each other. Make sure that you *keep talking* to each other about how you're both faring. Many couples do this as the last thing each night before they go to sleep.

- Make sure your partner attends to his own needs as well as yours and your family's. Don't let him burn out.

- Say "thank you" and "I love you" every day, not just to your spouse but to all those who are in this with you.

Use the support services offered by your hospital / cancer center and by organizations like the American Cancer Society and CancerCare. They have social workers and professional counselors for caregivers who are always available as well as caregiver support groups.

Your Parents

It doesn't matter that you're an adult; maybe you're a parent yourself or even a grandparent. But no matter how old you are, you'll always be Mommy's and Daddy's little girl—which is one of the many reasons it's so *especially* difficult to bring parents into the loop. There are few things more painful than having to watch one's child suffer a devastating illness.

Some people's relationship with one or both parents remains complicated long past childhood. If your mother was overprotective when you were a child, you shudder to think how she'll hover now. No matter what the nature of your relationship with your parents is, it will intensify as you fight this illness. To keep everybody in check:

- Remember that you're a grownup now. You can accept as much—or as little—help and/or advice from your parents as you want. And you can say, "No thank you" too.

- Stay honest. Your parents want to know the real scoop. Don't underplay what's going on in order to spare them. Remember, they're grownups too.

Your Children

If you have children, then you have yet another layer of concern to cope with. As most cancer-help organizations will tell you, the best thing you can do is tell your children what's happening to the degree that they're able to take it in and handle it. As you well know, children have great instincts, and yours are going to know early on that something's up. Just like adults, the less they understand, the more their vivid imaginations will take over and cause them to get more upset than if they were brought into the loop. It will be far better for them and for you if you tell them—sooner rather than later—and allow them to do things that will make them feel they're helping you get better.

The good news is that you don't have to go it alone. CancerCare, which offers many wonderful services, has a program called CancerCare for Kids. It's a staff of professional oncology social workers who offer you support and advice and will counsel your children to help them understand what's happening via telephone, online, or in person (cancercare.org; 800-813-4673).

CANCERCARE'S TEN TIPS FOR COMMUNICATING WITH YOUR CHILDREN

Give your children accurate, age-appropriate information about cancer. Don't be afraid to use the word *cancer* and tell them where it is in the body. Practice your explanation beforehand so you feel more comfortable. If you don't provide this information for them, they will often invent their own explanations, which can be even more frightening than the facts.

Explain the treatment plan and what this will mean to them—for example, Bobby's mom will be bringing them to soccer practice for a while. Prepare your children for any physical changes you might encounter throughout treatment such as hair loss, weight gain or loss, fatigue, and so on.

Answer your children's questions as accurately as possible and appropriately for their ages and prior experience with serious illness in the family. If you do not know the answer to a question, don't panic. Say, "I don't know. I will try to find out the answer."

Comfort your children by explaining that no matter how they have been behaving or what their thoughts have been, they did not do anything to cause cancer. Explain that they cannot "catch" cancer as they can catch a cold.

Let your children know about other members of the support system, including your partner, relatives, friends, clergy, teachers, coaches, and your health-care team. Let them know they can ask these adults questions and can always talk to them about their feelings.

Allow your children to participate in and make a contribution to your care by giving them age-appropriate tasks such as bringing a glass of water or reading to you.

Encourage your children to express their feelings, even ones that are uncomfortable. But also let them know it's okay to say, "I don't want to talk right now."

Assure your children that their needs are still important and that they will be cared for even if you can't always provide the care directly.

Spend your energy communicating with your children. Understand what they are asking even if you can't always provide the care directly.

As always, show them lots of love and affection. Let them know that although things are different, your love for them has not changed.

Friends, Strangers, and Answers to "How Can I Help?"

First, tell people how they can help. It sounds simple, but for many of us, it's very difficult to let others do things for us. If there's ever a time when you need to get over that, it's now.

It's very important to realize that other people really want to help you through this. And when they ask what you need, they mean it. You'll make it easier for them and for you if you're clear and specific about what would help you. If you need to make cupcakes for your child's class, ask somebody to do that for you. If you need someone to help you change your nightgown, ask a friend you're comfortable with. Trust me, if people aren't serious about being there for you, they won't ask again.

The next few pages are intended for you to make copies of and give to everyone who wants to help, including your spouse. Like all the information in this book, this information is the result of many people's experiences and is guaranteed to make your life a lot easier. Besides, by giving it to others, it will spare you from telling people things that are better conveyed by someone else.

Tried and True Ways to Help Your Friend

*It is one of the most beautiful
compensations of this life
that no man can sincerely try to help
another without helping himself.*

—Ralph Waldo Emerson

If you're reading this, then you're an important person in your friend's life. She has just been drafted into a battle for which she hasn't been trained. But she knows there are some people who will help her through this war, and you're one of them.

I've fought the same war, and I couldn't have done it without people like you who were there for me. During that time, I realized that just as I had no instruction manual for fighting my battle, my friends didn't have a manual to go by either.

Below are some guidelines for you as you help your friend. They're intended to help you keep from burning out too. After all, that's the best way to help your friend.

GOOD THINGS TO SAY

I'm so sorry this is happening to you.

I'm thinking of and praying for you every day.

You're going to get through this, and I'll be with you along the way.

When you're better (as opposed to "if you get better") . . .

Remember that you're *not* a statistic.

I can only imagine how hard this must be for you (not "I know how hard this is for you").

Please know that I'm here for you. Anytime you want to talk about anything, please let me know.

I don't know what to say, but I want you to know that I care.

WHAT NOT TO SAY

You're the last person I would have expected to get cancer.

What's your prognosis?

If you had to have cancer, this is the best one to get.

God is testing you.

RULE OF THUMB

Put yourself in your friend's place and imagine that someone was saying this to you. If it would make you feel better, then say it. If you wouldn't want to hear it, don't say it.

GOOD THINGS TO DO FOR YOUR FRIEND

Tell her—*don't ask* her—what you're going to do. For example, tell her that you're going to bring over dinner or a frozen casserole or schedule rides for her to and from treatments. You can always add, "Or is there something else that would be more helpful to you now?" This is much more helpful than asking the well-intentioned but less helpful open-ended question "What can I do?"

Bring food in disposable containers.

Call first. Any time you want to drop something off or visit, find out what would be a good time for you to come by.

Take your cues from your friend. She may want to talk about it a lot, or she may want to be more reticent. The main thing you can do for her is to let her know you care.

When you come by to pick up the kids and so on, *do not stay*—even for a cup of coffee—unless your friend begs you to.

If you do visit at her invitation, don't stay long.

Err on the side of too short rather than too long a visit. The gift of several brief visits is far better than that of one long one.

Don't be afraid to hug or touch your friend as you did before she was diagnosed. She won't break, and she's probably feeling pretty isolated by now and could use a good hug.

When in doubt, email instead of calling, especially if your friend doesn't have an answering machine.

Be sensitive about which books you give as gifts. Don't give or even recommend cancer memoirs unless your friend asks for one. Later on, she'll be more inspired by others' stories of overcoming their battles, but right now, she's busy fighting her own battle.

Don't tell your friend about other people you know who had cancer, even if they're better now.

Coordinate carpool rides for her children.

Drive her to treatments and offer to stay with her during treatment. You can probably go in and keep her company, which will not only comfort her but will also make the time fly.

Offer to care for her children when your friend has medical appointments.

Don't come to visit in groups, even as small as two people.

Send flowers with a note that simply says, "I love you." Or wait a bit and bring or send flowers later. There's never a bad time to receive flowers.

Celebrate milestones such as the end of treatment or when her hair starts growing back with a card or a small gift.

Don't give cream or lotion as a gift if your friend is having radiation; her skin will be sensitive to many ingredients in most of these products.

Consider waiting for a few weeks after her diagnosis or surgery before bringing her a get-well token or present. By then, the attention will have died down a little, and your gesture will mean that much more to her.

Keep your friend as involved and in the loop as possible. Include her in social events and projects. She probably won't participate much, but she'll feel as if she's still a full-fledged part of the group, and that's what's most important.

Don't offer unsolicited advice or opinions.

Don't spend time with her or her family if you have a cold or even the sniffles. Her immune system is pretty much gone.

Don't be patronizing. It's easy to slip into the singsong "so how's the patient?" mode. But that will make your friend feel even more helpless than she already does.

GIFTS GUARANTEED TO PLEASE

Never underestimate the value of a card! Send cards often throughout your friend's treatment. Buy a few at a time and address and stamp the envelopes so you can pop them in the mail frequently. No need for long notes—a simple "Thinking of you" works wonders. By the way, e-cards are nice, but nothing takes the place of ripping into an envelope that's just arrived.

Organize a card shower, which is just a fancy term for getting a lot of people to send cards. One email to as many of her friends and colleagues as you can locate is all it takes. Just be sure to include your friend's address. Since it's more fun to get cards on an ongoing basis than in one fell swoop, you all don't need to send them at once. When it comes to receiving cards, there's no such thing as too late.

Get her a subscription to a magazine she wouldn't normally get for herself, or if you have physical magazines, give her a few of your recent issues.

Give her a gift certificate to a local restaurant or bookstore or for babysitting services.

Combine the two above certificates to create a special time out of the house that she can use when she feels up to it. It will be an extremely welcome treat.

Offer to set up and maintain a page on caringbridge.com and write periodic health updates for your friend.

If you're paperwork-oriented, help with health-care claims.

Prepare a bag of goodies for your friend to take to appointments and treatment. Include such items as a magazine, water bottle, hard candy, pen and pad, and even a small pillow or microfleece throw.

Other great gifts you can give include little stones or medallions engraved with words such as *healing* and *serenity* or other uplifting words—I was given one and carried it in my pocket whenever I was out of my robe!—a pretty silk scarf square if your friend has lost her hair, music and meditation CDs, a prepaid long-distance telephone calling card, earplugs and an eye mask for sleeping, a small handheld fan with foam blades for the woman in menopause, a set of pretty blank note cards and stamps, or two hours devoted to doing anything she'd like done for her.

The internet offers all kinds of gifts, from chemo gift baskets—you can put your own together much more cheaply—to rubber cancer awareness bracelets to wear in support of your friend. These are listed at the back of this book. The more friends who wear them, the better.

But the best gift of all is simply being there and listening. There's no need to talk. Remember: you don't need to solve the problem. If you could, there'd be a Nobel Prize in your future.

Most important of all, don't take on too much. Since you're in this for the long haul, you need to make sure you don't burn out. Be sure to pace yourself so you won't disappear. It's far better to stay involved in a way that doesn't drain you than to exhaust yourself and become unable to continue to be there for your friend.

THINGS OTHERS CAN DO TO HELP THAT TAKE LESS THAN AN HOUR

Run the vacuum.

Take your kids out for ice cream for a change of pace for everybody.

Put a load of laundry into your washer.

Put a load of laundry into your dryer.

Straighten out the refrigerator contents and toss some if necessary.

Make some sandwiches, snacks, or lunches ahead for your kids.

Separate junk mail from your personal mail, magazines, and catalogs.

Help you make a list of people who have been sending things and helping you so you can acknowledge them after you're better.

Bring over a takeout lunch and share it with you.

Run a load of dishes in the dishwasher.

Unload the dishwasher.

Pick up your prescriptions. Make sure they take your insurance card.

7

Staying Home and Going Out

Regardless of your job situation, it's important to remember that *you have a new full-time job: you're a CEO.* Not only that, you aren't putting in an eight- or ten- or twelve-hour day; you're spending 24/7 on this job. And on top of everything else, you're doing all this with diminished energy and strength, not to mention those annoying things like nausea, loss of appetite, and anxiety. You're now working two jobs when it's harder than it was to do just one.

Not many of us have the luxury of taking an unpaid leave of absence, although many employers are legally bound to provide one for a designated period of time. If you have disability insurance, you may be eligible for short- or long-term disability benefits. Even if you think you know what the answer is, check with your employer. It would be a shame if you were to miss out on benefits you assumed you didn't have.

Staying Home

It sounds obvious, but do as little housework as possible. Don't straighten up when people visit; they aren't thinking about what your house looks like.

ATTRACTIVE HOME WEAR HINTS

Whether you're greeting company or just getting the mail, glance in the mirror before you open the door. Not to make sure you're wearing lipstick—or even your robe. I'm just trying to spare you from opening the door and then remembering, not necessarily right away, that you're not wearing anything on your baldhead. If, on the other hand, you don't want a return visit from that particular person, it's probably a good idea. Other hints are:

> Keep a scarf or cap somewhere near the front door so you can put it on at the last minute when the doorbell rings.
> Invest in a good robe and slippers. You'll be getting much more use out of them than almost anything else except your PJs—and not because you'll be

feeling so sick; you'll just want to be as comfortable as possible.

If you're entertaining guests at home and want to dress up, comparatively speaking, yoga clothes provide both comfort and style.

If you've been put into menopause thanks to your treatment, keep a couple of extra nightgowns by your bed since you may well want to change in the middle of the night due to the sweats.

ENTERTAINING VISITORS—WHO'S THE SICK ONE HERE?

People have the best of intentions, but they don't always know what isn't appropriate. That said, it is not your job to educate them or indulge them if you don't feel like accepting their visit right then. Your job is to rest, conserve your energy, and take care of your needs. You can be gracious and firm; they'll understand. If you're not up to having visitors, some things you can do include the following:

Just say no.

Use the good cop / bad cop routine. If possible, have your spouse or partner answer the phone or the door and say, "She'd love to see you, but she's resting."

Invest in caller ID. Use it to screen calls.

Feel free to ignore your email's instant messaging or check to see if you can change your availability icon onscreen. Some email programs let you set your availability as "busy."

Don't answer the door if somebody rings your doorbell unannounced.

When you're up for company, here are some things you can do to save energy and enjoy your visit more:

Pretend you're the guest. Try not to start fixing plates of cookies and cups of coffee for your company. They aren't here because they're hungry, and they certainly don't want to put you to work. If you feel you must offer refreshments, say something like "The tea bags are in the canister if you'd like to make yourself a cup."

Don't get dressed. Seriously. Stay in your PJs and robe if you want to make sure your guests remember just why they're there. It's a constant, silent reminder that your body is at war and it's tired.

Have an exit strategy. There's nothing worse than being ready for your guests to leave before they are. If you have your out planned in advance, you'll enjoy the visit much more knowing that you won't be needing to figure out a tactful way to say it's time to leave.

> Have an exit strategy. There's nothing worse than being ready for your guests to leave before they are.

When I was growing up, when company was staying a little too long, my father would address my mother and say, "Let's get to bed, honey, so these good people can get home." I opted for a less blunt approach. The best exit strategy I found was to tell my guests in advance that I was delighted they were coming, but I had an appointment and would have to end the visit at X o'clock. People will usually assume that your "appointment" is with a doctor, but in my case, it was often just with my down comforter and DVD player. But it was an appointment, right? This worked like a charm every time. I also realized that my guests were relieved to have an exit strategy too!

Making the Most of Going Out

During my treatment, I'd have been happy to stay home most all the time. Not because I felt so ill—I felt surprisingly well for most of it—but because my energy was definitely limited, and my bald head always required some attention. But how many of us have the option to stay in? I had to go to work, doctors' appointments, grocery shopping—in other words, life went on. Which is actually a good thing. After all, that's exactly what I was fighting for.

TIPS FOR GOING OUT

Rule of thumb: dress for yourself, not for others. If it makes you feel better to wear makeup and heels, do it. But if you don't:

- This is your chance to go casual. If you're still working, dress nicely, but you don't have to be a fashion plate. If you're going to someone's house for dinner, wear something comfortable. If there was ever a time when nobody's concerned about whether your shoes match your outfit, it's now.

- Piggyback errands you must do. Keep a running list of errands you need to do so that when you go out, you can be most efficient.

- Let others do errands for you; save your energy for the things you want or have to do.

- Ask a friend to drive you to do your errands. This is a great way to take advantage of people's offers to help. And think of all the energy you'll save just by not having to find parking spaces.

8

Top (Approximately) Ten Lists

THINGS TO DO WHILE WAITING

To see the doctor
Write thank-you notes.

To see the doctor again
Catch up in your journal.

To start your next round of chemo
Take up a crossword puzzle or sudoku.

For your next round of radiation
Start working on your holiday gift list; it's never too
early.

For a CT scan

Breathe a prayer for those who are there for you, doing their best to help make this all a little easier for you.

For a bout of nausea to pass

Sorry, I can't help you out there. Do whatever it takes.

For your prescription

Pretend you're being interviewed on national TV about what you're going through. Give your own advice for getting through cancer treatment with your sanity intact. Who knows? Maybe they'll invite you back.

To finish a round of chemo

Decide what you're going to treat yourself to after your next round of chemo. You know what you're treating yourself to after this one, right?

For your hair to grow back

Think about how you can thank the people who've been there for you after life gets back to normal—and remember that it will. You may want to have a tea after your treatment is over and give your guests a small token of gratitude.

For your ride

Nothing. Do nothing. Close your eyes, breathe, be still.

Music to Have Chemo By

Brandenburg Concertos 1–6, J. S. Bach

Piano Concerto No. 21 in C Major ("Elvira Madigan"), W. A. Mozart

The Best of the Capitol Years, Frank Sinatra

Duets: An American Classic, Tony Bennett

Kind of Blue, Miles Davis

We Shall Overcome: The Seeger Sessions, Bruce Springsteen

Songs of Hope and Comfort, Andrea Bocelli

Movies to Entertain and Distract

There's a reason the phrase "mind over matter" has been around for so long: it's true. I found that watching movies— as long as they weren't tearjerkers—was one of the best ways to take a mental break from my body. Here are some great ones.

FEEL-GOOD MOVIES

Barb and Star Go to Vista Del Mar

Mrs. Harris Goes to Paris

Hunt for the Wilderpeople

Bridesmaids

The Wizard of Oz

When Harry Met Sally

Grease

Sister Act

Annie
La La Land
Mamma Mia
Clueless
Moonstruck
The Birdcage
Elf

DRAMAS

The Secret Life of Bees
To Kill a Mockingbird
Butch Cassidy and the Sundance Kid
Because of Winn-Dixie
The Godfather I and *II*
The Help
Where the Crawdads Sing

COMEDIES

The Pink Panther (1963, starring Peter Sellers)
The Producers (1968, starring Zero Mostel and Gene
    Wilder)
Young Frankenstein
A Night at the Opera
Bringing Up Baby

MUSICALS

Little Shop of Horrors
The Phantom of the Opera

Guys and Dolls
Show Boat
Grease
Funny Girl

Novels to Make Time Fly

Memoirs of a Geisha, Arthur Golden
The Stone Diaries, Carol Shields
Anna Karenina, Leo Tolstoy (It's very long but is an
    incredible love story.)
The Gold Coast, Nelson DeMille
To Kill a Mockingbird, Harper Lee
The Good Earth, Pearl S. Buck
The Kite Runner, Khaled Hosseini
Where the Crawdads Sing, Delia Owens

Decide to Debunk Myths about Cancer

The following list was selected from authoritative sources, including the National Institutes of Health, the Mayo Clinic, and the American Cancer Society.

THE FOLLOWING STATEMENTS ARE FALSE:

Sugars feed cancer.
Nausea, sickness, and pain always accompany cancer treatment.

If cancer information is on the internet, then it's true.

If cancer information is on the printed page, then it's true.

If the lump hurts, it isn't cancer.

You can prevent skin cancer by applying sunscreen once every day.

Antiperspirants or deodorants can cause breast cancer.

Your attitude—positive or negative—may determine your risk of cancer.

Herbal products can cure cancer.

Cancer will always come back.

Everyone with the same kind of cancer gets the same kind of treatment.

Drinking coffee increases your chances of getting breast cancer.

Things to Remember When You're Really Down

This, too, shall pass.

You are *not* a statistic.

The day is coming when cancer won't dominate your thinking, time, energy, and life—really and truly.

You're not in this alone. You're surrounded by people who would do anything for you except probably take your place. But you can't blame them for that.

There are still things to be grateful for. Think of three.

A year from today, this will be behind you.

You're probably facing the hardest thing you'll ever have to deal with. So it can get only better from here.

Good Things That Will Happen as a Result of Chemo

When something goes wrong and you say, "It could be worse," you mean it.

No more hair on your legs, in some cases.

No more hair under your arms, in some cases.

Your skin will look like someone's who is twenty years younger than you.

You can say, "Sorry, I'm just not up to it," even if you are, for at least the next several months.

You will never take the hair on your head and eyebrows, nose hair, and pubic hair for granted again.

You'll never wish you didn't have an appetite.

You'll have a new level of compassion and understanding of others who are undergoing chemo.

You won't take everyday things for granted.

Thick, lush hair on your head will replace your old hair.

9

Complementary and Integrative Therapies

There was a time when the medical cancer community rejected nontraditional approaches to healing. But today, integrative therapies and complementary therapies are recognized for their value in the cancer world. Memorial Sloan Kettering Cancer Center and M. D. Anderson Cancer Center, the top two treatment centers in the country, both maintain integrative medical service departments, which offer a range of therapies from acupuncture to yoga.

Here are the terms to know:

Integrative medicine: An approach to medical care that combines conventional medicine with complementary and alternative medicine (CAM) practices that have been shown through science to be safe and effective. This approach often attempts to address the mental, physical, and spiritual aspects of health.

Conventional medicine / standard medical treatment: The system in which health professionals who hold MD or DO (doctor of osteopathy) degrees and use drugs, radiation, and/or surgery to address cancer. It is also known as mainstream or Western medicine.

Complementary therapy is used with conventional treatment but is not considered by itself to be conventional treatment. Acupuncture is an example, which is used to help lessen some of the side effects of cancer.

Complementary and alternative medicines are different from each other, even though they're often discussed in tandem. Alternative medicine is used *in place of* conventional medicine. Complementary or integrative medicine is used *together with* conventional/standard medicine. The American Cancer Society stresses that current scientific evidence shows alternative therapies *in place of* standard cancer treatments have much higher death rates.

Around half of all cancer patients use at least one CAM therapy during their course of treatment. Some of the most common complementary therapies include acupuncture, used for pain and nausea; healing touch; massage; yoga; meditation; journaling; guided imagery; reflexology; Pilates; tai chi; and dance, music, and art therapies. Integrative medicine uses therapies that include acupuncture, biofeedback, chiropractors, clergy, exercise trainers, herbal protocols, massage, music, pharmacologists, meditation and relaxation techniques, physical therapists, physicians who specialize in complementary and integrative medicine, physical therapy, and psychologists or psychiatrists.

Before you decide to take advantage of any CAM therapies, run it by your doctor to ensure avoiding any adverse effects or reactions due to interactions with your medical protocol. Find out if your health insurance covers CAM treatments. Most are not covered, so check out the costs in advance.

The American Cancer Society sanctions the following CAM therapies in conjunction with standard treatment:

- Acupuncture may help with mild pain and some types of nausea.

- Art or music therapy may promote healing and enhance the quality of life.

- Biofeedback uses monitoring devices to help control heart rate, blood pressure, sweating, and muscle tension.

- Massage therapy is often used to decrease stress, anxiety, depression, and pain.

- Prayer and meditation help many gain a sense of peace and confidence and reduce anxiety and fear.

- Tai chi and yoga have been shown to improve strength and balance.

Alternative medicine: While there are many benefits to complementary and integrative therapy, alternative medicine/therapy is something to approach with great caution. If you're considering using any method *instead of* standard medical treatment, the American Cancer Society urges you to:

- Be wary of any treatment that says it can cure cancer.

- Be wary of treatments that are only available in one clinic, especially if it is located in another country with less strict patient protection laws than the United States.

- Find out about the education and training of anyone who might treat you.

- Find out if clinical trials or scientific studies have been conducted on people, not just animals, and which side effects have been reported.

- Learn whether the findings have been published in trustworthy journals after being reviewed by other scientists.

RESOURCES FOR FURTHER INFORMATION

American Cancer Society—www.cancer.org / treatment types

National Cancer Institute—www.cancer.gov /
complementary and alternative medicine
National Institutes of Health—www.nih.gov / health
information

10

Survivor!

*Although the world is full of suffering, it
is also full of the overcoming of it.*
—Helen Keller

Saying Goodbye to Treatment

A funny thing happened on the way to finishing up my treatment. I began to get anxious. Actually, I started dreading my upcoming final treatment. As bad as the chemo and all that had gone with it had been, I'd had megadoses of ammunition and rays destroying the cancer cells in my body. Even when I slept, they were busy hunting down and

151

decimating the sinister cells that had invaded my body and my life.

Now I was about to be pushed off into uncharted waters by myself. A friend described it as feeling like a little row-boat being launched onto a lake without oars or a pilot—or an anchor. The other side of the lake was in sight, but suddenly it was up to me to get there by myself. I didn't want to row the boat alone.

When my doctor said, "I'll see you in three months," I wanted to beg him to let me come back before then. "How about if I come back in a few weeks, and you can freshen up my chemo?" I wanted to ask him, as if we were talking about a glass of wine.

Nobody was more surprised about these emotions than I was. I'd spent months that felt like years dealing with endless insults to my body and soul. But now that it was time to start to detox, I found myself afraid to say goodbye to chemo.

It was a big relief to learn that my feelings and fears were common. In fact, the American Cancer Society has found that many survivors are surprised by concerns and fears that they hadn't anticipated.

Not only is there a fear of being sent offshore without a rope but residual side effects of treatment are also probably still making you tired, even though you feel as though you need to go back to your normal responsibilities and routines. And there's also a nagging fear that the cancer could come back. But the brain is a beautiful thing, and these fears are going to recede until someday you'll wake up and you won't think about them for a few minutes. Then half an hour, a few hours, a day—pretty soon you realize you haven't thought about a recurrence for a week! Wonder of wonders, one day it occurs to you that you haven't thought about your cancer—or about cancer at all—for quite a while.

This is hard to imagine, I know. When I was in the throes of cancer, I couldn't believe that I'd ever get back to "normal" or that I wouldn't constantly be aware of the fact that cancer had once invaded my space. But I can honestly tell you that I hardly think about having had or getting cancer again except for when a scan is approaching. My life is full and active; I have fun, work, friends, family, hobbies, pursuits. It's . . . normal.

Normal. What a beautiful word. But don't rely on my word.

Am I different than I was before I had cancer? Yes. And I'm not saying that your life will be the same as before. It won't. Hopefully, you'll take fewer things for granted. You'll live more in the moment. Your priorities will probably have changed a little or a lot. You'll have a new appreciation for simple things, like being able to grocery shop without getting tired and walking for more than a couple of blocks. You'll have a special sense of empathy for and identification with those who are still members of the club—even strangers. If they mention that they have cancer, you won't cringe and remember that you have to be somewhere else. You'll ask what kind of cancer they have, and you'll let them know that you understand, that someday they won't wake up thinking about cancer, and that one day they'll have burned their membership cards too.

Everything I Need to Know I Learned in Treatment

> *Every day is a precious gift*
> *Don't waste today worrying about tomorrow*
> *Unconditional love is a joy to give and a blessing to
> receive*
> *There are no coincidences . . .*
> *God shines through the people we love and guides us*
> *Slow down*
> *Take deep breaths*
> *Believe in miracles*
> *Don't quit*
> *Never give up hope*
> *Doctors and nurses and their families are extraordi-
> nary people who need our prayers*
> *Prayer is powerful*
> *Everyone should spend at least one day in an oncolo-
> gist's office*
> *Be generous with your praise*
> *Say "thank you" often*
> *Don't allow little things to upset you*
> *We need very few material possessions to live and be
> happy*
> *Smile*
> *Appreciate the humor in life*

Hug those around you
Thank God for family and friends who carry you
    through the difficult times
Eat healthy foods
Walk
Take time to listen to children
Have patience
Listen to music; it's healing
Take one day at a time
Stay in the present
Trust in God

—author unknown, posted in a waiting room at
the Dana-Farber Cancer Institute

Glossary

Here is a group of basic cancer terms that you'll probably encounter. They're just a fraction of the four thousand terms defined in the comprehensive *Dictionary of Cancer Terms*, which can be found at the National Cancer Institute website: www.cancer.gov/dictionary.

Acute—Describes symptoms or signs that begin and worsen quickly but don't last for a long period of time; not chronic.

Adjuvant therapy—Treatment given after the primary treatment to increase the chances of a cure.

Alternative medicine—Practices used instead of standard medical treatments. Includes megadose vitamins, herbal preparations, acupuncture, massage therapy, magnet therapy, meditation, healing touch, and other spiritual therapies.

Analgesic—Drug that relieves pain.

Anemia—Deficiency of red blood cells.

Asymptomatic—Having no signs or symptoms of disease.

B cell—White blood cell that comes from the bone marrow. As part of the immune system, B cells make antibodies and help fight infections.

Benign—Noncancerous.

Best practice—In medicine, treatment that experts agree is appropriate, accepted, and widely used. Also called *standard therapy* or *standard of care.*

Blood cell counts—Test to check the number of red and white blood cells and platelets. Low red blood cell counts cause tiredness. Low white blood cell counts increase the risk of infection. Low platelet counts increase the risk of bruising and bleeding.

CAR T-cell therapy—A type of cancer immunotherapy treatment that uses the patient's altered immune cells to fight cancer.

Chronic—Describes a disease or condition that persists or progresses over a long period of time.

Clinical trial—Research studies that test new treatment and prevention methods to find out if they are safe, effective, and better than the current standard of care (the best-known treatment). Unlike other scientific studies, these employ human beings as subjects instead of animals or laboratory testing.

Cold therapy—A system used to apply cold to scalp, hands, and/or feet during chemotherapy to reduce side effects.

Combination chemotherapy—Treatment with drugs that kill cancer cells.

Complementary medicine—A form of alternative treatment that is used in addition to standard/conventional treatments. Generally not considered standard medical approaches. May include dietary supplements, megadose vitamins, herbal preparations, special teas, acupuncture, massage therapy, magnet therapy, spiritual healing, and meditation.

Edema—Swelling caused by excess fluid in body tissues.

Grade—The grade of a tumor indicates its probable growth rate and tendency to spread. It depends on how abnormal the cancer cells look under a microscope and how quickly the tumor is likely to grow and spread. Grading systems are different for each type of cancer.

Hand-foot syndrome—Condition marked by pain, swelling, numbness, tingling, or redness of the hands or feet. A side effect of certain anticancer drugs.

Hope—To expect with confidence. To remember that every cancer at every stage has been survived by someone. An essential for every cancer patient.

Hormonal therapy—Treatment that prevents or slows cancer cells from growing by taking advantage of the hormonal needs of these cells.

Immunotherapy—A type of cancer treatment that uses substances made by the body or in a lab to boost the immune system and help the body find and destroy cancer cells.

In situ cancer—Early cancer that has not spread to neighboring tissue.

Invasive cancer—Cancer that has spread beyond the layer of tissue in which it started and is growing in other tissues or parts of the body.

Killer cell—White blood cell that attacks tumor cells and body cells that have been invaded by foreign substances.

Lesion—Area of abnormal tissue. A lesion may be benign or malignant.

Localized—Restricted to the site of origin, without evidence of spread.

Localized cancer—Cancer that is confined entirely to the area where it started and has not spread to other parts of the body.

Local therapy—Treatment that affects cells in the tumor and the area close to it.

Lymph, lymph fluid—Clear fluid that travels through the lymphatic system and carries cells that help fight infections and other diseases.

Lymph glands, lymph nodes—Pea-size organs that are located throughout the body. They filter out foreign substances and produce antibodies. Lymph glands filter lymph and store lymphocytes (white blood cells).

Lymphedema—Swelling in the arms or legs caused by excess fluid collected in tissues. It occurs after lymph vessels or lymph nodes are removed or treated with radiation.

Malignant—Cancerous; describes cells with a tendency to spread to other organs.

Margin—Edge or border of the tissue removed in cancer surgery.

Clean margin / negative margin—Terms used when a pathologist finds no cancer cells at the edge of the tissue, suggesting that all of the cancer has been removed.

Positive / involved margin—Terms used when a pathologist finds cancer cells at the edge of the tissue, suggesting that all of the cancer has not been removed.

Metastatic—Describes cancers that spread via the blood or lymphatic system to other parts of the body to form secondary tumors.

Millimeter—Measure of length in the metric system often used to measure tumors. There are twenty-five millimeters to one inch.

Mucositis—Complication of some cancer therapies in which the lining of the digestive system becomes inflamed. It is often seen as sores in the mouth.

NED (no evidence of disease)—Also referred to as *complete remission*. When all tests and scan results fail to find any cancer cells.

Negative test result—Test result that does not indicate the specific disease or condition for which the test was being done.

Neoplasm—Another word for tumor.

Neuropathy—Condition that causes numbness, tingling, burning, or weakness. It usually begins in the hands or feet and can be caused by certain anticancer drugs.

Neutropenia—Abnormal decrease in the number of neutrophils, a type of white blood cell.

Patient advocate—Person who helps a patient work with others who have an effect on the patient's health, including doctors, insurance companies, employers, case managers, and lawyers. A patient advocate helps resolve issues about health care, medical bills, and job discrimination related to a patient's medical condition.

Port—Implanted device through which blood may be withdrawn and drugs may be infused without repeated needle sticks.

Port-a-cath—Another term for a port.

Positive test result—Test result that reveals the presence of a specific disease or condition for which the test is being done.

Primary tumor—Place where the cancer first started to grow.

Protocol—Outline or action plan for a treatment program.

Radiation therapy—Use of high-energy radiation from X-rays, neutrons, and other sources to kill cancer cells and shrink tumors. Also called *radiotherapy*.

Radical mastectomy—Surgery for breast cancer in which the breast, chest muscles, and all of the lymph nodes under the arm are removed. Doctors consider radical mastectomy only when the tumor has spread to the chest muscles.

Refractory cancer—Cancer that does not respond to treatment. Also called *resistant cancer*.

Regimen—Treatment plan that specifies the dosage, schedule, and duration of treatment.

Regional—In oncology, describes the body area right around a tumor.

Regression—Decrease in the size of a tumor or in the extent of cancer in the body.

Remission—Decrease or disappearance of signs and symptoms of cancer.

Resected—Removed by surgery.

Resistant cancer—Another term for refractory cancer.

Response rate—Percentage of patients whose cancer shrinks or disappears after treatment.

Second-line therapy—Treatment given when initial treatment doesn't work or stops working.

Sentinel lymph node—First lymph node to which cancer is likely to spread from the primary tumor. When cancer spreads, the cancer cells may appear first in the sentinel node before spreading to other lymph nodes.

Stage—Extent of a cancer in the body. Staging is usually based on the size of a tumor, whether lymph nodes contain cancer, and whether the cancer has spread from the original site to other parts of the body. There are four stages: Stage I is localized, small, and easily treatable. Stages II and III are incrementally further developed. Stage IV cancer has spread to other organs, with surgery no longer being an option.

Staging—Performing exams and tests to learn the extent of the cancer within the body, especially whether it has spread from the original site to other parts of the body.

T cell—Type of white blood cell that attacks virus-infected cells, foreign cells, and cancer cells. T cells also produce a number of substances that regulate the immune response.

Tumor—Abnormal mass of tissue that results when cells divide more than they should or do not die when they should. Tumors may be benign or malignant.

Tumor marker—Proteins and other substances in the blood that indicate the presence of cancer cells somewhere else in the body.

White blood cells—General term for the cells in the body that play a major role in battling infection.

Resources

Services That Provide Help along the Way

There are scores of terrific nonprofit organizations whose sole purpose is to provide a huge array of amazingly generous, useful, free services to people with cancer and their families. Here are a few extraordinary ones.

American Cancer Society
Hope Lodge (www.cancer.org; 800-ACS-2345)
More than thirty facilities in the United States offer free, temporary housing facilities for cancer patients undergoing treatment along with their caregivers. Provides a supportive, homelike nurturing environment, run by the American Cancer Society.

Look Good, Feel Better (lookgoodfeelbetter.org)

Volunteer beauty professionals lead small in-person groups and virtual workshops, sharing techniques for skin care, nail care, makeup techniques, and options related to hair loss.

CancerCare (cancercare.org/1-800-HOPE)

Provides counseling with an oncology social worker, online workshops from leading oncology experts, help with navigating financial issues and securing proper care, and free publications.

Cancer Hope Network (cancerhopenetwork.org)

Confidential one-on-one peer support for survivors and families. You are matched with a trained volunteer who has recovered from a similar cancer.

CaringBridge (caringbridge.org)

Provides free, easy-to-create personalized websites. You can keep friends and family informed, and they can visit and leave messages. Available in all fifty states.

Patient Advocate Foundation (patientadvocate.org)

National nonprofit organization that works as a liaison between patients and employers, insurers, and creditors to resolve insurance, job discrimination, and/or debt crisis matters relative to their diagnosis. Its state-by-state financial resource guide lets you locate assistance for seeking relief from many illness-related expenses, from medication to food and utilities.

Red Door Community

Formerly known as Gilda's Club. Offers support groups for patients and caregivers, even posttreatment groups.

The Wellness Community (www.thewellnesscommunity.org)

Wonderful online support groups, nutrition information, mind/body exercises, and education.

Magazines

Coping with Cancer (copingmag.com; 615-791-3859): nineteen dollars for six issues per year. PO Box 682268, Franklin, TN 37068–2268.

Cure (curetoday.com); free subscription
National Cancer Institute (cancer.gov)
Offers dozens of patient education publications in a variety of formats
on topics including childhood cancer, clinical trials, coping and
support, screening, survivorship, treatments and side effects, and
specific types of cancer.

Retreats and Camps

Camp Make-A-Dream (campdream.org; 406-549-5987)
Free medically supervised retreats for individuals and families affected
by cancer. All services except travel are free. Includes kids camp
(ages six to twelve), siblings camp, and teen camp. Also offers
retreats for women, families, teens, and caregivers. Located in
Gold Creek, Montana. Open all year.
First Descents (firstdescents.org; 303-945-2490)
Offers outdoor adventures for young adults ages eighteen to forty-
five impacted by cancer. Includes kayaking, rock climbing, and
surfing in a variety of locations in the United States.
For Pete's Sake Cancer Respite Foundation (takeabreakfrom
cancer.org)
Provides a six-day stay with private accommodations at Woodloch
Resort in the Pocono Mountains. Free of charge to adult cancer
patients ages twenty-one to fifty-five and their caregivers and
children. Available to residents of Delaware, Pennsylvania, New
Jersey, New York, and Maryland.
Hole in the Wall Gang Camp (holeinthewallgang.org)
Free camps located in Connecticut and Maryland for children with
serious illness and their families.
Mary's Place by the Sea (marysplacebythesea.org; 732-455-5344)
Offers overnight and day retreats, free of charge. Located steps away
from the ocean in quaint Ocean Grove, New Jersey, ninety
minutes from New York City. Offers women in treatment or
up to two years posttreatment services that complement their
medical treatment, including oncology massage, individual
counseling, guided meditation, Reiki, yoga, and more.

Reel Recovery (reelrecovery.org)

Conducts free small group fly-fishing retreats for men living with all forms of cancer, led by professional psychosocial facilitators and expert fly-fishing instructors. Locations range from Maine to California.

Visit cancer.net and use the search function to find a more extensive listing of camps and retreats offered to those affected by cancer.

Online Supplies and Gifts

Choose Hope (choosehope.com; 888-348-4673)

Terrific catalog offering cancer-related items, from apparel—including my personal favorite, "Cancer Sucks" T-shirts, caps, and pins—to jewelry, caps, and even a "Cancer Daze" chemo care package and a Radiation Skin Care Bag. It also offers "queasy drops" hard candies. Started by a cancer survivor, Choose Hope donates 10 percent of its gross sales to cancer research.

TLC Catalog (tlccatalog.org; 800-850-9445)

Offered by the American Cancer Society. Reasonably priced wigs and related items. Also offers a range of mastectomy products.

Best Overall Cancer Websites

These websites are not in order of preference; they are all excellent and offer different types of services and information.

American Cancer Society: cancer.org
Association of Cancer Online Resources: acor.org
CancerCare: cancercare.org
Cancer Support Community: cancersupportcommunity.org
Dana-Farber Cancer Institute: dana-farber.org
Mayo Clinic: mayoclinic.org
MD Anderson Cancer Center: mdanderson.org
Memorial Sloan Kettering Cancer Center: mskcc.org

National Cancer Institute: cancer.gov
Patient Advocate Foundation: patientadvocate.org
Red Door Community (formerly Gilda's Club): reddoorcommunity.org

Cancer Awareness Colors

All cancers: Lavender
Bladder: Yellow
Bone: Yellow
Bone marrow transplant: Green
Brain: Gray
Breast: Pink
Breast (Male): Pink and blue
Cervical: Teal and white
Childhood: Gold
Colon and colorectal: Dark blue
Endometrial: Peach
Esophageal: Periwinkle
Gall bladder / bile duct: Green
Glioblastoma: Gray
Head and neck: Burgundy and ivory
Kidney: Green or orange
Liposarcoma: Purple
Leukemia: Orange
Liver: Emerald
Lung: White
Lymphoma: Lime
Melanoma: Black
Multiple myeloma: Burgundy
Ovarian: Teal
Pancreatic: Purple
Prostate: Light blue
Sarcoma/bone: Yellow
Uterine: Peach

For Further Reading

EVERYTHING HAPPENS FOR A REASON: AND OTHER LIES I'VE LOVED, Kate Bowler

Serious, funny, wise, searingly honest. Praised everywhere from *Real Simple* to the *New York Times*, this book, by a survivor of stage-four colon cancer, will make you feel like you have a sister who has been through the fire and is sitting alongside you sharing hard-won observations, crying beside you, and laughing beside you. If you only read one book on this list, read this one!

GETTING WELL AGAIN, O. Carl Simonton, MD; Stephanie Matthews-Simonton; and James Creighton

This classic walks you through the fear, confusion, and questions that accompany cancer and provides exercises and information to help you cope with and manage difficult issues in a positive manner.

CANCER VIXEN: A TRUE STORY, Marisa Acocella Marchetto

Everyone I know who has read this—including me—will tell you that once you pick up this book, which is done in a cartoon format, you can't put it down. It's written and illustrated by a successful Manhattan cartoonist fashionista who's engaged to a hot New York City restaurateur when she learns she has breast cancer. A big soul, lots of courage, great friends, and an amazing, irreverent sense of humor get her through.

WHY I WORE LIPSTICK TO MY MASTECTOMY, Geralyn Lucas

This memoir proves that humor is a major part of overcoming the horrors of cancer. The author shares her struggles with her sense of sexuality and self-image and what she learned on her own when she couldn't find guidance on how to cope.

LOVE, MEDICINE AND MIRACLES, Bernie Siegel, MD

A positive reminder that attitude plays a large role in moving through illness to health.

HAPPINESS IN A STORM: FACING ILLNESS AND EMBRACING LIFE AS A HEALTHY SURVIVOR, Wendy Schlessel Harpham

A physician and three-time cancer survivor shares the guidelines she has developed for getting through cancer. A sensible, realistic guide that illustrates how to cope with the fallout from serious illness and still nourish joy.

THE BREAST CANCER BOOK: A TRUSTED GUIDE FOR YOU AND YOUR LOVED ONES, Johns Hopkins Press

An authoritative, comprehensive, down-to-earth guide to organizations, support groups, websites, books, and videos. Everything you need to know in order to make the best decisions about diagnosis, treatment, and follow-up care.

Children's Books

WHAT HAPPENS WHEN SOMEONE I LOVE HAS CANCER?, Sara Olsher

Help kids understand more about what's happening when their loved one has cancer.

A good way to allow young ones to ask questions and help them through their anxiety. With her messy pigtails and sunny personality, young Mia and her stuffed giraffe help kids feel safe at a scary time.

Provides the knowledge that you're not alone, information about cancer, and a place for children to write down questions for parents, doctors, and teachers and draw pictures that represent their feelings for later discussion. Ages seven to twelve.

BECAUSE SOMEONE I LOVE HAS CANCER: KIDS' ACTIVITY BOOK, American Cancer Society

Support, encouragement, and information for children ages six to twelve. Creative activities allow your child to work through unfamiliar feelings and learn to recognize and tap into positive moments.

Complementary and Integrative Medicines

AMERICAN CANCER SOCIETY'S GUIDE TO COMPLEMENTARY AND ALTERNATIVE CANCER

METHODS, SECOND EDITION, American Cancer Society

The American Cancer Society reminds us that not all nontraditional methods of treating cancer are created equally. This is an up-to-date comprehensive volume with expert contributors who examine the evidence, both pro and con, for more than two hundred treatment methods.

CHOICES IN HEALING: INTEGRATING THE BEST OF CONVENTIONAL AND COMPLEMENTARY APPROACHES TO CANCER, Michael Lerner

Contains thorough discussions and evaluations of complementary programs—spiritual, psychological, nutritional, and pharmaceutical—as well as other less conventional approaches. Although the author believes that all people with cancer should be under the care of an oncologist, he provides a wealth of information that helps to clarify the overwhelming amount of data on alternative treatments.

General

AMERICAN CANCER SOCIETY CONSUMER GUIDE TO CANCER DRUGS, SECOND EDITION, Gail Wilkes

Explains cancer drugs to nonprofessionals and lists side effects and precautions for more than two hundred cancer-related medicines.

AMERICAN CANCER SOCIETY'S GUIDE TO PAIN CONTROL: UNDERSTANDING AND MANAGING CANCER PAIN, REVISED EDITION, American Cancer Society

There are lots of pain relief options, and there's no reason for you to live with unnecessary pain. Simple, invaluable information on how to work with your health-care team to create a plan that balances pain relief and the potential side effects of pain medications.

HELP! SOMEONE I LOVE HAS CANCER: HOW YOU CAN REALLY MAKE A DIFFERENCE, Joel Hughes

What do you say? What do you do? Through hard-won experience, Joel Hughes shares practical information and tools to help you navigate cancer with your loved one in ways that are truly supportive.

THE CAREGIVER'S GUIDE TO CANCER: COMPASSIONATE ADVICE FOR CARING FOR YOU AND YOUR LOVED ONE, Victoria Landes, LCSW

Practical advice from a licensed social worker for supporting your loved one while also practicing self-care.

WHEN A PARENT HAS CANCER: A GUIDE FOR CARING FOR YOUR CHILDREN, Wendy S. Harpham

The author—a mother, physician, and cancer survivor—draws on all of her experiences to teach parents how to help their children cope with the fears and life-changing demands that cancer places on everyone in the family. Includes an illustrated children's story, *Becky and the Worry Cup*, that illustrates the concerns kids have and ways to address them.

Puzzle Solution

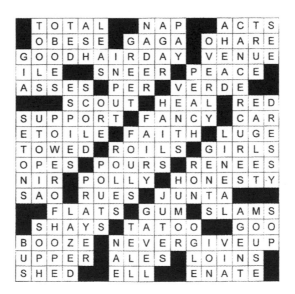

Acknowledgments

This book would not have been possible without my editor and champion, Adrienne Ingrum. She is not only an extraordinary editor, but also an extraordinary friend. Her colleagues at Broadleaf Books are accomplished professionals who have made the publishing process a pleasure. My thanks go to all of them and to Rachel Reyes and Jessica Lockrem, who guided this manuscript to finished book with grace and skill. Special thanks to Art Director Carlos Esparza for his brilliant cover design.

My doctors have literally saved my life. My deepest thanks to Dr. David Berman, who found something suspicious and would stop at nothing until he determined what the problem was. My oncologist, Dr. Michael Levitt, is brilliant, compassionate, dedicated, reassuring, and a team player who listens with care and acts with excellence. Finally, my thanks to Dr. Daniel Landsburg, who oversaw my CAR-T treatment. These doctors have extended my life by years. How can I ever thank you?

I have the best friends in the world. My deepest gratitude to them for their amazing encouragement and support throughout the years. They include Lynn Appelbaum, Andrea Doering, Anthony DeStefano, Jordan DeStefano, Tobi Graff, my sister Joan Kowal, Liz Leahey, Katherine McEneaney, Susanna and Tom Schindler, Lucia Tasker, Andrea Weinzimer, Rebecca and Lance Wood, and my grandchildren, Summer and Dan Wenzl.

Many thanks to Abbie Wood, the first to share her wisdom with me to ease my own cancer journey.

Index

About the Author

B.C. (before cancer), Michelle Rapkin would have told you all about her work. Now, however, she knows better. While she has enjoyed a career in book editing and writing, her most important descriptors are friend, wife, sister, stepmother, and grandmother.

She lives at the beach in Ocean Grove, New Jersey, with her beloved dog, Maxie.